Holy BARIATRIMONY

Christopher White

Holy Bariatrimony
Copyright © 2016-2020 Christopher White

ISBN: 978-1-7341945-1-7 (Paperback Edition)
ISBN: 978-1-7341945-0-0 (Ebook Edition)

www.holybariatrimony.com

ACKNOWLEDGMENTS

Special Thanks:

Above all, to my wife **Patricia**, for keeping me focused,
disciplined, and inspired

To **President George Bush, Senior**
For signing the **Nutrition Labeling and Education Act of 1990**
(which requires nutrition labels on packaged foods)

To **President Barack Obama**
For signing the **Patient Protection and Affordable
Care Act of 2010**
(which requires calorie information on restaurant menus)

To **Dr. Thomas Sonnanstine IV and Team**,
Patty's bariatric surgeon
For a surgery more successful than they could imagine

To **Drs. David DeWalt** and **Jennifer Rittenberry**
For diagnosing and treating my diabetes

To **Albert Lee, Mike Lee,** and **Under Armour**
For the **MyFitnessPal suite of smartphone applications**
Which became an indispensable tool in our journey

To the **National Weight Control Registry**
for adding my name to its groundbreaking research study

To **Mindy McGinnis**, whose advice and direction led to the
publication of this book
(www.mindymcginnis.com)

To **Jill Di Donato**, my editor, and author of *Beautiful Garbage*
(www.jilldidonato.com)

To **Stephanee Killen**, interior book designer,
and author of *Buddha Breaking Up*
(www.integrativeink.com)

To **Romana Bovan**, cover designer

Books That Inspired Me

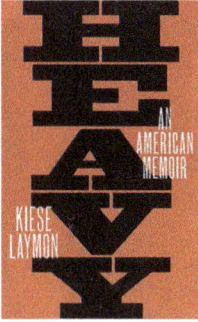

Heavy
by Kiese Laymon

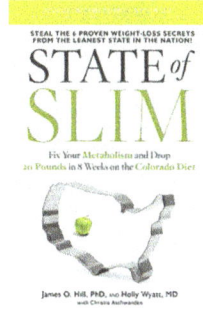

State of Slim
by James Hill
and Holly Wyatt

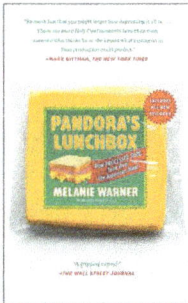

**Pandora's
Lunchbox**
by Melanie
Warner

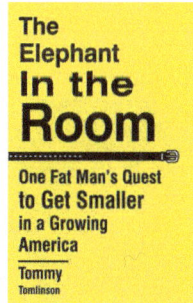

**The Elephant in
the Room**
by Tommy
Tomlinson

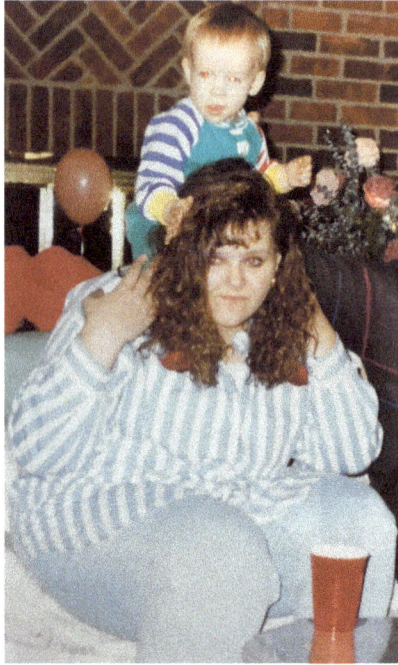

Patty & Chris in the early 1990s, soon before they met.

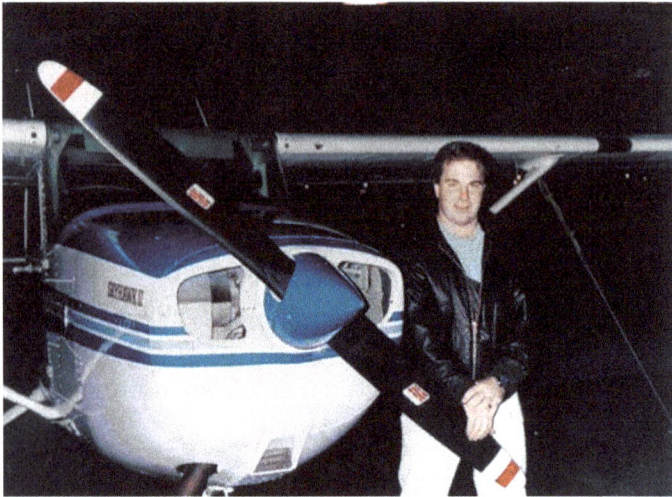

INTRODUCTION

$\mathcal{I}$t happened in the late summer of 1998. I was taking classes at Ohio State's Fisher College of Business, and I got a text message from my fiancé, Patricia. Patty told me that she saw a TV ad for an upcoming concert. Amy Grant was planning a Christmas music tour, and was coming to our hometown of Columbus, Ohio, on December 10, 1998. Patty urged me to get tickets, because she really wanted to go.

I was a poor, broke college student, grumbling about the cost, but didn't want to fail my new fiancé, so I ordered the tickets.

When the evening of the concert arrived, we found a parking spot not too far away, though the walk was not very comfortable. We arrived at the Schottenstein Center, the cavernous arena where the Ohio State Buckeyes play their home basketball games. The usher directed us to our section, so we could take our seats.

In this case, however, our seats could barely take *us*.

These were basketball-arena seats. They were designed for teen-something or twenty-something college kids. Patty and I were a bit older. I was 33, and Patty was soon to be 29. But our age wasn't the real problem. It was our weight.

1

Together, we weighed north of 600 pounds. We managed to live our lives in such a way that we weren't reminded of our size every day, but during special occasions, like a concert in a basketball arena, we got a reality check. Patty's hips were too wide for the seat. She struggled to wriggle her way into her seat, but no matter what she did, she could not get comfortable. Before the concert even began, she started to complain. Her hips were sore. Her back was *very* sore. Her legs were getting numb. And she was embarrassed. I felt awful for her. A concert was a rare occasion for us, and I wanted her to enjoy it. I told her I would go ask an usher if we could move to a handicap seat, but she stopped me, even though she was crowding the person on the other side of her, and miserable, and unable to enjoy the concert.

On that evening, Patty resolved to be smarter when we go to an event like that. She resolved to only get seats on the end of an aisle. She resolved to get seats in the front row of a section, so people could get past us. And, above all, on that evening, like many before and many since, Patty resolved to lose weight.

As a school-age kid, my *own* weight was not much above normal. I played summer sports, and often rode my bicycle around Cardington, the small Ohio town where I spent my childhood. At age eleven, I got a newspaper route that kept me on my bike for several miles per day. However, when I received my driver's license at the age of sixteen, I slowly started putting on weight. In college, I had a round belly and a full face. I needed ever-bigger clothes. I earned a pilot's license in 1991, a process that required a medical exam every other year. During that decade, the aviation doctor often mentioned my weight and that I needed to lose some. But it didn't keep me from passing the physical, so there was no urgency.

And that lack of urgency was a problem. Although I was heavy, it didn't seem to affect my life very much. I wasn't suffering insults, and I didn't have any noticeable pain. I *did* manage to lose some weight when I tried to, such as when a girlfriend broke up with me in 1992 and I lost about 40 pounds as a result. But, my sedentary habits returned, and so did the weight. At my peak, in 2009, I weighed 291 pounds, and I stayed about that weight until the middle of 2012.

Patty, whom I married in 2000, had been vexed by her weight since her pre-adolescence. She *did* suffer pain, *and* the insults. As a child and teenager, she was called "Two-Ton Tessie," and "Elephant." I started dating her when she was 25, and despite her youth, she often complained of back pain. Occasionally, her pain would be so severe that I had to take her to the emergency room for treatment.

But, my, she was a wonderful cook! When we started dating, she would bring plates of food to me at work. Her lasagna was magnificent. I had no idea of the calorie load, and I didn't care. It was just so tasty, and it made my co-workers jealous.

She also made the most heavenly double-layer pumpkin pie ever. Each Thanksgiving, Patty made her signature pumpkin rolls for her family and friends, and sent a few to work with me. My co-workers would *fight* over these pumpkin rolls. For the Christmas season, she would make hundreds of cookies for everyone to share, as well as her chocolate-covered Oreo truffles, which were another crowd pleaser. I could eat these by the dozen, and I did. The evidence was in *both* our waistlines.

She *always* wanted to lose weight. She did constant research, and she seemed to be an expert at weight loss, except at how to make it apply to *herself*. She joined weight-loss challenges with her friends and shed a few pounds. But she always regained them. I remember cautioning her about losing a lot of weight, because there's always a danger of gaining it all back and then some, and that would be worse for her health than just staying big and beautiful. Plus, I didn't really want to diet along with her. She had an apathetic husband who didn't see our weight as that much of a problem. So what if we couldn't go to concerts or basketball games? So what if we had to buy clothes online? So what if we had to buy heavy-duty furniture? We were happy. We enjoyed food, and we were healthy enough.

Until we weren't.

I went to see my family doctor in late 2012. After looking over my bloodwork, he came out and said it. And finally, he had my attention.

I had diabetes.

I was 47 years old, and my body wasn't going to be as forgiving of my eating habits as it had been when I was younger. I had never really cared how I looked, but my health *was* important to me. He recommended small, sustainable changes rather than a sudden transformation to my behavior. Among the first changes he urged me to make was in my soda intake. He said rather than drinking regular soda, I should drink half-regular and half-diet, and then increase the percentage of diet soda until the regular stuff no longer appealed to me. I was skeptical, but I tried it. And over the months, it worked. I also ate more salads and less pizza. I stopped putting dressing on my salads, which actually made them seem more filling.

My weight slowly came down. By the end of 2013, I had lost about 15 pounds without really trying. And I never gained it back.

All this made Patty feel even worse. She continued to struggle with her weight, and wouldn't even tell me how much she weighed, except to admit that she was well over 300 pounds.

One day, at our son's flag-football game, the boys were receiving their trophies and were standing in line while their moms took their team photo. In a fit of whimsy, I took out my phone and decided, instead of taking another photo of the team, that I would take a photo of the group of moms while *they* took photos of the team.

Later, I showed Patty the photo I took. Instead of the chuckle I was expecting, she thrust the phone back at me and ordered me to delete it. As tears welled in her eyes, she exclaimed, "I'm so tired of being the *fat* Mom!!" I was speechless, and I marveled at the disconnect between the affection with which I looked at her, and the disgust with which she looked at *herself.*

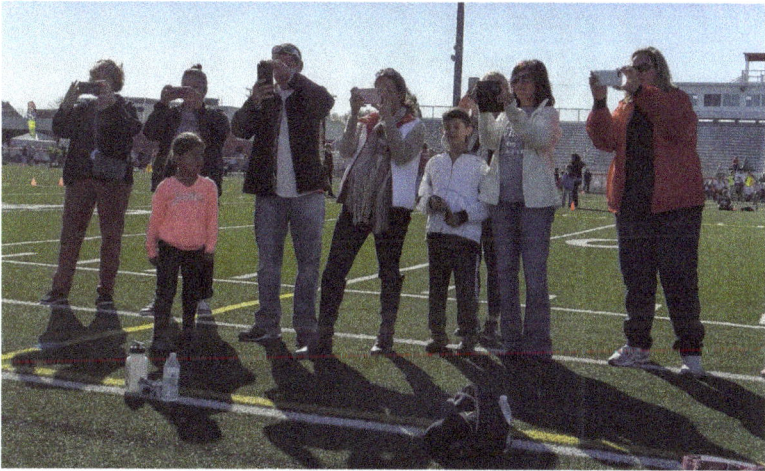

Patty's "Fat Mom" photo

She started researching this miracle cure called 'bariatric surgery'. She read websites and joined bariatric Facebook groups. She appealed to her doctors to help her convince our insurance to cover this procedure.

But, I knew there was no way it would be covered. From what I'd seen, bariatric surgery was for people who were morbidly obese; people who couldn't breathe, who needed power scooters to get around. People who would literally die without it. My wife was different. She was beautiful, capable, and outgoing. She juggled three kids and a house, and a large family with two parents and three sisters and their nine children between them. All of them lived in our city, and rarely a day went by without a visit from some of them. She was always on the move, and in my mind, the last thing she needed was bariatric surgery.

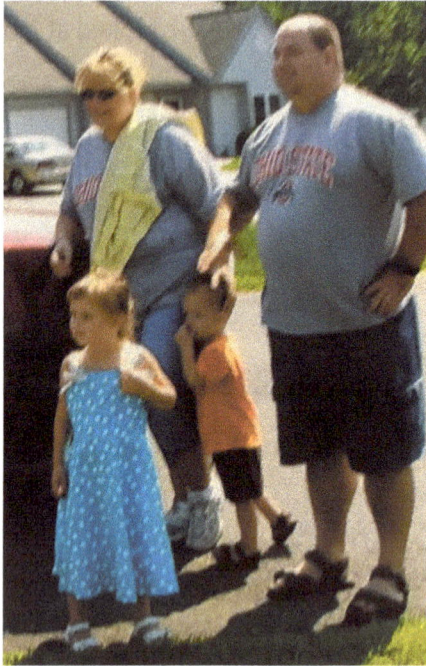

Chris & Patty with Kaitlyn(3) and Kyle(2) in 2007. Patty was pregnant with Nicholas. Chris was pregnant with complacency.

Plus, I had another concern about this surgery. Not a medical concern, but a relationship concern. I read blogs like ObesityHelp and MyBariatricLife, and the stories were alarming. Stories abound on how cracks in the marriage are laid bare as the pounds go down. I learned that divorce is very common among couples when one partner undergoes this surgery. The last thing I wanted was a bariatric divorce.

I actually began to look at this surgery as a threat to our marriage. I was sure it wouldn't be approved, and I secretly *hoped* it wouldn't.

Patty, for her part, kept up her dogged persistence. As I predicted, her surgery got denied. But she scoured the appeals process. She enlisted the help of her doctors, and had them write letters. She studied other patients' stories online for any angle she could use to be successful. She saw this as her only salvation, and she threw herself into it, through rounds of applications, denials, and appeals, until one day the post office delivered a unicorn.

An approval letter.

I read and re-read the letter in disbelief, and even a little terror. Holy Bariatrimony, I thought: *This is actually going to happen!*

I started re-reading those blogs. I tried to tease out how much the husband's reaction to the wife's weight loss contributed to the breakdown of the marriage. But these stories were so one-sided. I was never able to get the *man's* side of the story, and I found that frustrating.

Patty had a few months to prepare for the surgery. She was supposed to lose a little weight on her own, about 10 pounds, before they could operate. She had to get some specialized bloodwork, and wait for the results. She had a new slate of doctor appointments to keep, and she had to plan how the kids and I would manage for the few days she was to be in the hospital.

I read some more. I was excited for Patty, but also fearful of the future. There were a couple of ways I could navigate this. The path of least resistance was essentially to do nothing. I didn't have to change *my* lifestyle; all the changes were going to be on *her* end. I read that bariatric surgery is not always successful, especially long-term. People sometimes gain all that weight back, and it turns out to be a huge waste of money. It was easy, and tempting, for me to just dismiss this whole thing as another ineffective weight-loss boondoggle, just like all the other ones she had tried, while I smugly make myself yet another plate of nachos.

Or, I could commit to a different path.

I love my wife. Completely, to my core, I love her. Patty and I have been together for more than twenty years, and in that time, she has validated me as a man like no other. She accepted my ring, she took my name, she bore my children. I *owe* her this. I really *want* her to succeed. And deep down, I know that *my* reaction will play a major role in how successful she is.

What would the future be like with a slim wife? Would she be healthier, happier and more confident? It was terrifying to think of Patty as a new woman, one I'd never met. But at the same time, I was filled with excitement over the unknown. There are lots of stories on marriages dissolving over weight loss, but I was determined not to be one of them.

Yet, on these blogs I was reading, there was a frustrating lack of guidance for guys in my situation. I will have to write that guidance for myself.

If I'm going to keep our marriage strong, I'm going to have to adapt. I'm going to have to change my *own* habits, as well. The many changes this surgery will *force* on her, are the same changes I'm going to have to *choose* to adopt for myself.

My first decision is this: I will not fear this surgery. I will not try to talk her out of it; I will not try to prevent it. I'm going to support it, and I'm going to support Patty through it. This is going to be the biggest challenge of my married life, and I'm going to do what I can to meet it. She will not travel this road alone. I will stick right by her. Step by step, and day by day,

I will make it my mission to join her on this life-changing, unpredictable journey.

And my mission begins...*today.*

NOVEMBER 2016

Tuesday, November 29, 2016

Surgery day. It went as expected, no complications. I saw Patty after she was assigned to her room. She was woozy and had plenty of belly pain from the gas they used to inflate her abdomen.

Afterwards, I picked up our 13-year-old daughter Kaitlyn from cheerleading practice, and went home to relieve my mom from babysitting our two sons. I emptied the dishwasher, and folded the last of the laundry. I let the kids eat whatever sweets were left in the house...Lord knows they're not going to see much in the way of junk food in the house anymore.

The kids are being pretty good, and not giving my mom too much of a headache. Patty was worried about how they would react to her being gone for a few days, but so far, it seems they're taking it just fine.

Wednesday, Nov 30, 2016

I got the kids up and off to school on time. After they were gone, I brought an airbed into the living room so our boys,

Kyle (11) and Nicholas (8), could sleep on it tonight with their grandma next to them on the sofa. I'll be at work until after midnight, so I expect them to be asleep when I get home.

Patty called me around noon; she sounded better, and her voice was louder. She had been up this morning walking laps around the hospital floor. I had a free hour in the afternoon, so I was able to go to the hospital to see her. I walked laps with her. Of course, she had already made friends among the nurses and staff. I've always admired that about Patty, how she can make friends out of strangers so naturally. I could never really find things to talk about like she can...for her, it's effortless. I helped her back into bed and plugged in her high-tech IV pole.

The boys were *not* asleep when I got home, but I was told they had napped in the evening while I was gone. I've got to get them up for school in five hours. Yay for me!

DECEMBER 2016

Thursday, December 1, 2016

*P*atty came home today! She called me from the hospital in the late morning to come and pick her up. I waited out front for her, and I was expecting her to be wheeled out in a wheelchair, but no....She *walked* out of the hospital, accompanied by a nurse carrying Patty's bag. For someone who had surgery two days before, she looked awesome. She was in a good mood, and looking forward to going home.

In the past, when I brought her home from the hospital, she always wanted to go to a drive-thru and get a Coke and something to eat. But, today, she didn't even mention it. She said she had some Jell-O and a little broth in the hospital and was feeling stuffed. So the changes, in terms of food, have started immediately.

I felt proud of myself when we walked in the house together. I had picked up the kitchen and the living room and I felt the place looked pretty good for her arrival. Nothing was out of place, everything was wiped down, and I tried very hard not to leave a mess to stare her in the face when she got home.

Her first words when she walked into the house were, "Why does it stink in here?"

Friday, December 2, 2016

Can you say exhaustion? For two days in a row, I've gone to bed at 2 a.m., and gotten up at 6 a.m. to get the two older kids off to school, then woke up the youngest kid to get him ready and out to the bus...then I got called out to work a 16-hour day before I even had a chance to brush my teeth. I spent the entire day in a slow-motion fog.

This morning, I went to the Speedway gas station to refill my diet soda. I do not remember paying for it. They probably watched me walk out with an 85¢ drink in a zombie-like stupor, and they probably laughed. They know me. I'm sure they'll razz me about it next time I'm there.

Patty is trying to adjust to her new food reality. She is making some milkshake-thingy with yogurt and protein milk and some sort of powder. She asked me to buy banana-cream pudding mix tonight so she can add it to her shakes. She's also drinking beef broth. She's on a liquid-only diet for a couple of weeks to allow her stomach sutures to heal without getting particles of solid food in them.

Saturday, December 3, 2016

I slept today. Boy, did I sleep today. At least ten hours, and then a half-hour nap before work. I feel so much better.

Patty is having trouble with her milkshakes. It seems that anything with milk in it is giving her diarrhea. She's drinking more broth instead. It's too bad that she can't eat rice and toast and bananas that can typically help with stuff like that.

She sent me to the store tonight for soup, and Cream of Wheat, and unflavored protein powder. I couldn't find the powder. I might have to go tomorrow to a nutrition store to find it.

Sunday, December 4, 2016

We need more blenders. We have two, and they are getting one heck of a workout. Patty is blending everything she eats (or, rather, drinks). Butterscotch pudding with protein powder and whipped cream (very good). Cream of Potato soup (not so good). She made baked fish and french fries for the kids and me (delicious).

Monday, December 5, 2016

Less than a week post-surgery, and Patty has started to exercise. Today, she walked 30 minutes on our treadmill. This is the $900 treadmill she made me buy two years ago that I said she would never use, and for two years, I was right. Today, she made me wrong. She walked at 2 mph at zero incline. (When I use it, I walk at 2.8 mph at a 5% incline.)

I went back to the gas station today for a soda refill. I told the clerk that I didn't pay for the one I got on Friday. He rang up two drinks for me. Then the register printed out a coupon for a free one. So, karma has smiled on me today.

When I got home, I sat next to Patty on the couch, and she had her hand on my knee. She told me, "Don't get any skinnier... you're getting bony." I said, "Seriously? You're about to lose the weight of two people, and you're telling *me* not to get skinnier?"

We're going grocery shopping tonight. It will be interesting to see what she decides to bring into the house.

We're back from the grocery store. She bought a lot of instant oatmeal for the kids and me. She also got herself some sugar-free popsicles. No chips, no soda, no snack cakes, no cookies. The kids are going to start complaining in the coming days. Too bad.

Tuesday, December 6, 2016

"Maybe I'm just fat, and *supposed* to be fat." Patty is moping today. After losing ten pounds the first week, she gained back six. She weighed herself last night before bed, which is wrong... the other times she weighed herself in the morning. She's been drinking water, or Powerade, all day. So, she put back on some of the water weight. She talked to her doctor today, and she was told to quit worrying and she is doing just fine.

Tonight she made spaghetti and meatballs for the kids and me, and she had a chocolate protein milkshake. I'm really going to have to ask her what she puts in those shakes.

Wednesday, December 7, 2016

Patty went out grocery shopping today. She is getting back into more of a normal routine. She was gone in the afternoon, which allowed me to take a quick nap, and I missed her text message. She had wanted me to meet her at the store, but I slept through it.

I had some tomato soup and a bowl of rice, which is too many carbs for me. It was a cold day, and the food was comfy. But comfort food does not really lead to comfort, at least not long term. I'll finish what we have, but then I'm not going to buy any more of that stuff.

Thursday, December 8, 2016

Patty went to the middle school for 11-year-old Kyle's choir concert tonight, and she got in a lot of walking. She lost her Fitbit, so she doesn't know how many steps, but her sore back tells her it was a lot.

She has a hard time drinking all the fluids and protein she is supposed to. She blended up some cream of potato soup today, but couldn't finish it. She says she gets too full and feels nauseous.

She's cold. She's been complaining about getting chilly since the surgery. A few nights ago, I had to steal an extra blanket for her from the boys' bedroom. Because of her post-surgery chills, I got her a new electric blanket this week as an early Christmas present. Now, she's much happier at night.

There is a cold snap this week, with wind chills near zero, and I was out working in it. Patty was in bed when I got home, so I asked her to crank up my half of the blanket to high, so it will be warm when I went to bed. There are few feelings like coming in from the bitter cold and crawling into bed with your wife under a toasty electric blanket. It's like pulling up to a parking meter with an hour still on it, or finding M&M's in your mailbox. It's unmitigated joy.

Friday, December 9. 2016

I kept forgetting her diet guidelines, so I had to ask her again. During the liquid-only phase of her post-op diet, she's supposed to drink 64 ounces of fluid, and consume 60 to 80 grams of protein per day. She also challenged me to do the same thing. I said I was committed to doing this with her, so I'll try.

She *is* getting a little thinner. I can see it in her face and neck. This morning, after she got the kids off to school, she came upstairs and climbed into bed with me. She gently shook me awake. She asked, "Have you been called out to work yet?" "Nope," I replied drowsily. "Not yet."

"Hmmm…"

Then she gazed at me with *those* eyes. And with *that* smile. Her wordless directive; her way of letting me know that we were about to share a milestone moment.

So, this morning, ten days after her bariatric surgery, Patty and I made love. It was slower, and more gentle than normal, but she reported no pain or discomfort, and afterwards, she displayed the glow that I've been missing so much. I'm sure this is medically important information, right? And it sure is great to have my wife back!

Afterward, she slept in until the early afternoon. Maybe it's that new electric blanket that keeps her in bed. I doubt it's me.

Saturday, December 10, 2016

Laundry. Lots of laundry today. One of the boys wet his bed last night, and so he retrieved several blankets and piled them on top of the wet bed, then laid on the blankets. I guess he was comfortable, but it only caused all of those blankets to become dirty laundry, on top of the normally high piles of laundry our family of five generates. We have two washers and two dryers in our basement laundry room, but it is still going to be a lot of work on Patty. She told me she had more than 16 loads to do after sorting through all the clothes.

I brought home a pound of chocolate covered raisins, that I was planning on putting into my Cream of Wheat for tomorrow's breakfast. But instead, I ate the whole pound while watching YouTube early in the morning. I have a weakness for chocolate covered raisins, but I've really got to ignore cravings like that. If I force myself to write about my transgressions in this journal, then maybe I can better resist them.

Sunday, December 11, 2016

Patty is still having a hard time consuming 60 to 80 grams of protein, per doctor's orders. At bedtime, she's only had 29 grams. I can feel her silent frustration.

Our treadmill is in the basement in the laundry room. While she walked on the treadmill, I kept her company folding the laundry. Our youngest son Nicholas turns nine tomorrow, and Patty was making cake pops for him to share with his class. She hasn't been making treats like that lately. She used to share dessert recipes on Facebook, but she doesn't anymore.

I shouldn't take credit for folding the laundry. It was just a couple of blankets. She has been doing laundry nonstop for the last two days, and she's down to three or four loads. For a stay-at-home mom, Patty outworks everyone I know.

The quote of the day goes to 11-year-old Kyle. I told him to make his bed, with the new sheets and blankets that Patty just washed, and I promised him he'll be very comfortable and will sleep soundly.

"I'm not going to sleep soundly...I'm going to sleep soundless!"

How do you correct a boy who's more correct than you are?

Monday, December 12, 2016

Patty is getting really tired of the liquid diet. She's trying to drink all of the protein but is really craving solid food. She says she'd give anything to eat an egg. She's looking forward to her next appointment in a couple of days, hoping her surgeon will give her the green light to eat soft solids like mashed potatoes or Cream of Wheat. She made *me* a bowl of Cream of Wheat, with some protein powder, brown sugar and raisins. It was fabulous. She has always been a great cook, and I'm worried that since she won't be eating a lot of the great food she makes, she'll start losing her cooking skills. That might sound chauvinistic of me. I guess I could learn to cook my own damned self.

I'm reading a book called *Deep Down Dark*, about the 33 Chilean copper miners who were trapped in a collapsed mine for two months in 2010. After 2½ weeks, the men were near starvation when a drilling team finally completed a six-inch hole into their refuge. But they couldn't send food to the starving men right away, because their bodies were so weak a sudden feast could kill them. Instead, they sent down little bottles of glucose gel to recondition their stomachs.

I think of that book when I see my wife with her tumbler of protein shake, which she sips with a grimaced face. But until her stomach heals from surgery, she can't eat solid food, because it could kill her.

Tuesday, December 13, 2016

It snowed a few inches today, and I got some exercise shoveling the driveway and the sidewalk. Patty made dinner: shrimp and broccoli for me, and puréed chicken noodle soup with protein powder for her. She also made some chicken and mashed potatoes for the kids and she was very tempted to eat some of the potatoes. I told her, "No way. I don't want to take you to the emergency room in the snow and cold."

She is frustrated that she is not losing weight more quickly. I told her, "You don't want to lose weight too fast. You'll look like a deflated airbag, hanging limply from the steering wheel…"

Wednesday, December 14, 2016

Patty braved a very cold morning for her two-week doctor appointment today. She was told she was doing great. Apparently, the most rapid weight loss occurs in the heaviest people, and Patty, at just over 300 pounds, was by no means the heaviest.

The food restrictions are a little more relaxed now. She doesn't need as much protein, and she told me on the phone that she was looking forward to having an egg and some cottage cheese today. I thought, 'better you than me.' Yuck!

Thursday, December 15, 2016

Patty did a lot today. Running nine-year-old Nicholas to the speech coach and then to school, taking my mom out shopping for groceries and Christmas, housework, laundry, cooking, gathering trash for the curb. I hope she didn't overdo it. But I admire her sense of mission. You just can't keep her down.

Friday, December 16, 2016

She overdid it. Big time.

Patty woke up this morning in pain. Back hurting, stomach hurting, everything. She ate some pureed chili yesterday, and she's wondering if she has gas pain due to the beans. She took one of her pain pills, which she usually avoids if she can stand it, and she sent me to the store to get Milk of Magnesia.

She announced that she is staying in bed all day, and the housework will have to wait. I shrugged, kissed her, and went to work. We had lots of freezing rain tonight, and thick ice was covering everything. A co-worker ripped the door handle off her car trying to get in it. I'm glad Patty is home in bed; that's the safest place to be tonight.

Saturday, December 17, 2016

Patty is feeling better today, but still not great. And she still gets chilly. We're having a cold snap this week. The days are very short, and this weekend we've had freezing rain and fog. Patty has had the fireplace on and has been sitting on the couch, covered with a blanket.

I slept late and when I came downstairs she made me eggs and shrimp. An unusual brunch, but a high-protein one, and that's how she is cooking now. Low carbs, and high protein. I tell her that she has become a Protein Preacher.

11-year-old Kyle is quite the special case. He loves junk food, and he loves to hide somewhere while eating it. We often find boxes of Cocoa Puffs and Apple Jacks behind the couch, or a jar of Nutella hidden behind the toilet, or empty cans of soda under his bed. When he is not hiding somewhere, he is boisterous and loud and a prankster, and likes to annoy his siblings. So, sometimes when he disappears somewhere else in the house, we can assume he's eating something. But we like the peace and quiet so much that we just let him be.

However, since the surgery, Patty is bringing less junk food into the house, and Kyle is finding his options to be more limited. This weekend, Patty found a bar of baking chocolate behind the couch, with only a couple of bites taken from it. As enraging as this sounds, it might be an improvement. He apparently didn't like it, so he abandoned it. And it means he had nothing else more appealing to squirrel away. Baby steps.

Sunday, December 18, 2016

Patty is in a good mood today. She got up out of bed this morning and headed to the bathroom. Then she climbed back into bed and woke me up. She had checked her weight. For the first time in many years, she has broken the 300-pound barrier. She weighed in at 298. She finally admitted her starting weight to me; it was 317 on surgery day. She would never tell me before.

In those lazy minutes before getting up, she lay on her back next to me, and I lifted her T-shirt so I could caress her bare breast. I told her, "You know, you're going to lose these…"

She laughed, and said, "No, I'm not! Just a little bit."

"Nah…they're going to be teeny-tiny."

"Oh, are you going to leave me because my boobs get smaller?"

"Of course not. It will be exciting…Like I'm having an affair…"

She yanked her T-shirt back down.

Our son Nicholas turned nine this week, and today was his birthday party. It was at a trampoline and swingset store that hosts birthday parties in their showroom and allows the kids to play on their showpieces, hoping to entice the parents to buy them.

I really have to hand it to my wife. She can plan a birthday party for a nine-year old-boy that draws at least 26 people, on a freezing cold Sunday after an ice storm, only one week before Christmas. She is absolutely amazing. If I tried to do something like that, I would get a couple dozen polite declines.

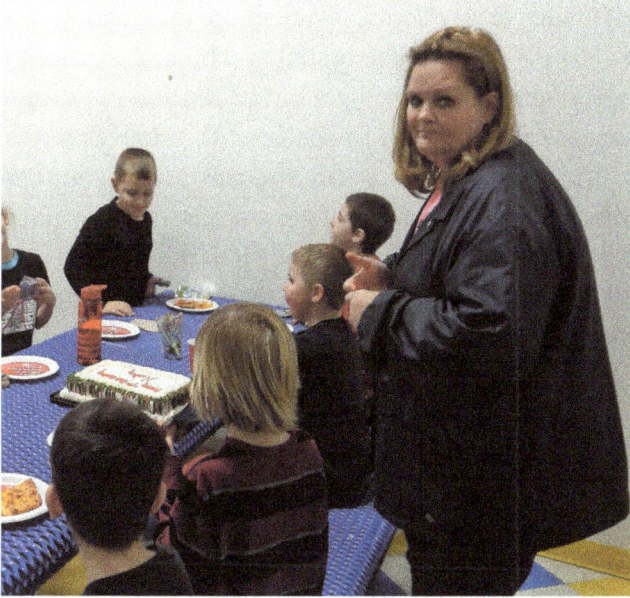

Patty, in charge of Nicholas's birthday party

Monday, December 19, 2016

Patty is really tired today. She was still fighting chills, but we found out one reason...our thermostat was set to only 62 degrees. She didn't do that, and I didn't do that...so one of the kids must have fiddled with the thermostat. We reset it to the mid-70s, but the house does not seem that much warmer. Patty is sitting on the couch, wrapped up with a blanket. I just got another blanket and I'm about to join her.

She doesn't know yet that I'm writing this journal, and that's why I can be as candid as I am. If she was editing it every day, it wouldn't be *my* journal; it would be *ours*.

She ran the gas tank in her minivan almost dry this week-end, and she was worried about taking the kids to the bus stop this morning without running out of gas. She was talking to me about it when we were both awake in the middle of the night. I decided to be a hero, and go on out and fill up her van. It was in the single digits outside, so I got out of bed and put on a t-shirt, and hooded sweatshirt, and a coat, and then a stocking cap and gloves. The gas station was only two miles away, but I wanted to be ready in case I ran out of gas on the way. I would have a cold walk home. Fortunately, I made it to the gas station. I filled the tank and came back home. She smiled and hugged me and had my electric blanket warmed up for me to return to bed. Then, in the morning, she brought me breakfast in bed: eggs and sausage. It's the little things, I guess. She can be too easy to please sometimes. (But, not usually.)

Tonight, we watched my favorite Christmas movie, *Mercy Mission: The Rescue of Flight 771*. We found it free on YouTube and cast it to the living room TV through our TiVo box. She loved it. Now it's *her* favorite Christmas movie, too.

Tuesday, December 20, 2016

Patty is still struggling with the constipation and the stomach and back pain. She thought she might even have a kidney stone. She's even been talking about going to the hospital, but today was the last day of school for the kids before Christmas break, so her sense of maternal duty will probably keep her home.

Work was light today, so I got home early. This afternoon, I took her minivan to Valvoline to get the oil changed and the low tires filled up. During this cold snap, I've been complaining about parking my own van out on the street and having to defrost it each morning, while Patty's van is snug and warm in the garage. She drives the older kids to the bus stop during cold mornings about 90 minutes before I get up, so it makes more sense for her to have the garage. I still complain about it though. Since the kids are off school for the next two weeks, Patty offered to let me have the garage during break. That's when I felt like a jerk for complaining about it. I declined, mostly because the cold snap is about over and it's going to be in the thirties and forties during the next few mornings.

Dinner for me was fish and garlic mashed potatoes. We cooked the fish in the air fryer, the new appliance she got last month. She's been experimenting with it. She didn't eat any of the fish, but she *did* have some of the mashed potatoes.

After I ate, she asked me how I liked my cauliflower.

"Huh? I didn't have cauliflower. You made me fish and potatoes."

She gave me an impish grin.

"Those weren't potatoes, were they?," I asked.

She made garlic mashed cauliflower that I just *assumed* were potatoes. They were good! And creamy! Like mashed potatoes! Except they had much fewer calories and carbs.

Score one more for Patty.

Wednesday, December 21, 2016

Still constipated. Still frustrated. Still talking about going to the hospital. Still talking herself out of it.

I found out today that, after 16 years of marriage, I'm apparently eating yogurt the wrong way. Patty and I buy the Dannon Light and Fit Greek Yogurt; she likes the solid flavors like strawberry cheesecake and blueberry. I like the kind with the fruit on the bottom, especially cherry. Today, Patty got a cherry yogurt out of the refrigerator for me, opened it, and mixed it up before handing it to me. I shouted, "NNOOOOOOOOOOO!!!!!!!"

She recoiled. "Wha...Wha...WHAT?!?!"

"You mixed it up! I don't like that!"

"But, that's how you're *supposed* to do it!"

"No! I like the eat the plain yogurt on top before I get to the cherries on the bottom!"

She made a contorted, disgusted face, as if I had just told her I like to eat landfill sludge. "Oh, my God, Chris, that's gross!"

Our 13-year-old daughter Kaitlyn chimed in, "Dad, that's disgusting!"

Since when did the women in my family become the yogurt police? I don't care. I'm going to eat *my* yogurt *my* way. The girls can mix up their own damned yogurt. I feel better already.

Thursday, December 22, 2016

She still tires easily. She did some more Christmas shopping and grocery shopping because the kids are now on their holiday break from school.

I've been concerned about how she is feeling, and haven't paid much attention to myself. My throat started getting sore yesterday, and today I have a full-blown throat infection. It was so bad, I had to leave work early. I don't get sick often, but when I do, Patty says I act like a baby about it. So I have *that* to look forward to. Hopefully I'll feel better tomorrow.

Friday, December 23, 2016

I feel worse. After spending the morning in bed, Patty ordered me out of bed and over to urgent care. The doctor confirmed my throat infection and gave me prescriptions for amoxicillin and an antihistamine cough syrup. I didn't want to go to the doctor. I'm glad I did.

Saturday, December 24, 2016

I felt well enough to make an attempt at going to work. It was going to be a short shift because it's Christmas Eve, but I couldn't even finish it. I was only at work for an hour before I came home.

Patty and the kids went to her sister's home for their family Christmas gathering, while I stayed home to recover. Patty didn't cook all the goodies that she has in previous years; she only made some buffalo chicken dip. When she got home, she told me that the kids were complaining there was nothing there to eat! It hadn't dawned on her that in the past, she was bringing most of the food to these gatherings, and without her baking marathons, the table was bare.

Sick or not, Santa has to work, so when we finally got the kids to sleep, I wrapped and tagged presents and stuffed stockings and sent the Elf on the Shelf back to the North Pole by way of a storage tub in the crawl space. Our youngest is the only one that still believes this charade, so maybe these Christmas Eve nights will get easier in the future? No, I don't think so either. At 5 a. m., I went back to bed.

Sunday, December 25, 2016

The kids slept in today. This is very out of character for them on a Christmas morning. We got to sleep until 10:30.

Patty made biscuits and sausage gravy for brunch. We had six guests from extended family come by, in addition to our own family of five. My sister Amy brought a fruit salad, which was actually more popular than the biscuits and gravy.

Patty has lost 19 pounds so far, three-and-a-half weeks in. She is complaining that she can't see the weight loss in her figure yet. I've noticed it in her face and neck, and others have too. But she tends to wear baggy clothes, so it's not so apparent anywhere else.

I've lost a single pound, mostly because I haven't felt well enough to eat anything. I *do* feel better, though. The throat pain is gone. Now, I'm just dealing with a persistent cough and feeling tired.

Patty was a little daring today; she tried some bread. It was a small piece of a sub bun that she wrapped around a bigger piece of ham. She also made some hot chocolate with whipped cream. Afterward, she had a bellyache, which she had to deal with the rest of the evening and into bedtime. She's really being a grump, too. I contribute to that, because sometimes when I'm tired (or bored) I'll sneak upstairs and nap, and that can infuriate her. (And I've been very tired these last few days). Of course, other husbands just park themselves onto their recliners, instead. I've never owned a recliner, and I never will...I want to live my life on my feet.

Also, the kids open their gifts and play with their new stuff and leave messes, and that makes her mad, too. These kids really need chores.

Monday, December 26, 2016

Patty had some energy today, and we were all worse off for it. She wanted to work on the basement, which meant clean and vacuum, and to have me set up the Xbox One the boys got for Christmas. Of course, we were to do this whether we wanted to or not, and we didn't want to. We did anyway, because Patty was militant about it. When she gets on a cleaning mission, it's difficult to be in her presence. So, the kids opted to close themselves in their rooms. She even complained about it on Facebook.

I'll hand it to her, the basement *did* look pretty nice after it was done. But I didn't enjoy the process one bit.

Tuesday, December 27, 2016

Patty took the kids to the YMCA and talked to a trainer there about a family exercise program. I'm very skeptical about it. My theory is that you cannot *force* another person to get healthy, even your own kids. You could be a source of leadership and inspiration, but the drive has to come from within. Plus, our schedules would never work. Our 13-year-old daughter Kaitlyn is a middle-school cheerleader, so she gets her conditioning at after-school practice each day. Our nine-year-old son Nicholas loves to swim, so that's what he will do when he is at the YMCA. The one that needs more exercise is our 11-year-old son Kyle, and he's pretty stubborn. I don't think he will get interested in his health and appearance until he gets interested in girls. But, we shall see.

Patty is still complaining of chills, and she's not able to drink all the fluids she is supposed to drink each day. She just fills up too quickly. And she said her urine is deep yellow and smelly, which she believes is due to dehydration. She did a half-hour on the treadmill today, and was able to drink a bottle of water during that workout.

Wednesday, December 28, 2016

Patty sure gets cold easily. She shivers under blankets, and tells me to feel her nose...which feels just fine to me, but then she dismisses my opinion by telling me my hands are cold. She wears a jacket in the house; she drinks hot Carnation Instant Breakfast, but she just can't shake the chills. She says it's a common complaint after bariatric surgery. But she doesn't like it. I went upstairs and turned on her blanket, so she'll have a happy surprise when she goes to bed.

I ate a chopped salad with dried cranberries, nuts, and apple slices. She watched me eat it with envy in her eyes. She can't have lettuce or other raw vegetables yet. After two months, she can have a salad. She says she is craving a chicken salad from Chipotle Mexican Grill, and she'll treat herself to one after her two-month anniversary. I responded, "Wait a minute...You're planning to celebrate an accomplishment with...*food*? I thought we were over that now. Food isn't a celebration, it's a problem. Remember?" So, it looks like the surgery doesn't really stop the cravings. It just prevents one from acting on them.

She just climbed into bed, and called down from the bedroom, "My husband's awesome!" That blanket heated up quickly.

Thursday, December 29, 2016

One month post-surgery. Patty has lost 20 pounds. She says she'll lose 20 more next month. I disputed that with my husband-y wisdom. "Weight loss is not linear. You might lose more than 20...you'll probably lose less."

We have a bet now.

She complains about her belly. It hasn't gone down as much as she wants. I don't know what to tell her. I think she's beautiful, but hearing it from me doesn't impress her.

Friday, December 30, 2016

Patty did some more treadmill walking today. Otherwise, nothing new to report.

Saturday, December 31, 2016

I went to an endocrinologist today to go over my blood-work. I've lost another 14 pounds since August, and my A1C was a normal 5.6 (seven months ago, it was 10.5). In fact, *all* of my numbers were normal except for HDL, which was 29. It should be 40 or above, but it improved from the 26 it was in August. The doctor suggested more exercise (of course) and a fish oil supplement. It was a good visit.

Patty slept late today. I left the house at 8 a.m. and got home from the doctor and a short day of work at about noon, and Patty and the kids were still in bed. It was fine by me; a sleeping wife gives no orders. I crawled back into bed next to her, and slept until 4 p.m. She was up by then.

She was despondent tonight. She is feeling tired and lethargic. She's saying she regrets having the surgery. She isn't losing weight fast enough. She doesn't think she will lose anything going forward. She's also depressed about the Fiesta Bowl tonight, where our Ohio State Buckeyes got blown out by the Clemson Tigers 31-0.

She's been binge-watching *The Fosters* on Netflix these past few days. Patty watches it in the living room, and Kaitlyn is watching the same show in her bedroom. Patty is mad at our daughter for getting her hooked on this show. Patty also likes a broadcast show called *This Is Us*. There is an overweight couple on there, and the woman has decided to have bariatric surgery. I should probably watch it, but I haven't watched TV in decades, probably. I love to read, and listen to podcasts and audiobooks. According to Goodreads.com, I've read 50 books this year. Patty has read two. She's much more of a television fan.

JANUARY 2017

Sunday, January 1, 2017

elcome to the New Year. I'm looking forward to it. This will be the most dynamic year of our marriage. That could be good, or it could be bad. I'm determined to make it a good one.

Patty is going to lose a *lot* of weight this year. She will be a very different woman. I expect her to experience much less pain. I expect her to feel much more confident. I expect her to be much more assertive, with her sisters, with her parents, with our kids, and even with *me*.

I want to take some family trips this year. We have two large amusement parks in Ohio: Cedar Point on the Lake Erie shore, and Kings Island near Cincinnati. We go to Cedar Point every spring, on a day reserved for alumni from Ohio State University. That's a blast, and we love it. I plan to do it again this year. 30 years ago, I *worked* at Cedar Point. I was young and single then, and the memories this annual trip brings back are a source of joy for me, and a source of frustration for Patty and the kids, as I blather on and on about days gone by.

As a family, we've never gone to Kings Island, and I want to change that this year. Both trips involve a lot of walking, which Patty has struggled with because it hurts her. This year, that is going to be different, and I'm very hopeful about it.

I also want to visit the Ohio State Fair this summer. It's held right here in Columbus, but for some reason, we have never gone there as a family, probably for the same reason, all the walking. I hope to change that this year, as well.

We went to the zoo tonight. The Columbus Zoo has its Wildlights each holiday season, and this was the final night of this year's event. We were there walking around for about 90 minutes, and Patty's back was starting to get sore. I was hoping that one of the benefits of this surgery was to reduce her back pain when walking, and maybe her endurance has improved with the weight loss she has already achieved, but we're not quite there yet. We all had a terrific time anyway, and I'm glad we went with our kids.

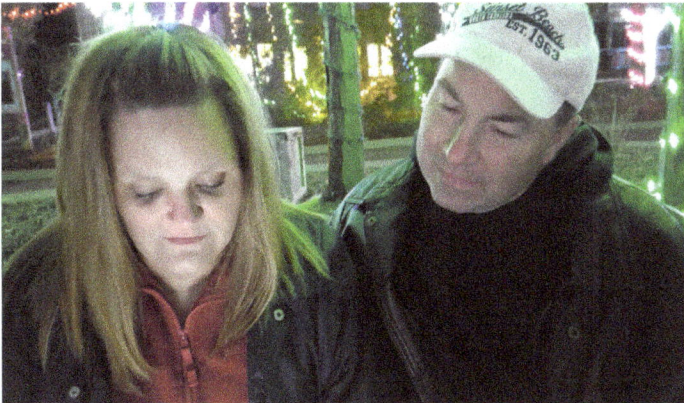

Patty & Chris at the Columbus Zoo Wildlights

Monday, January 2, 2017

We slept late. The kids have one more day of vacation before they return to school. Last night, the kids and I had a funnel cake at the Zoo, and I wondered if they could be made at home. We looked up the recipe and it was dead simple, so Patty made a few funnel cakes this afternoon in a pan of canola oil. She, of course, did not have any, but I had a couple, and they were very tasty. But I got over my craving, and didn't ask her to make any more tonight like she had planned.

We had our parents over for dinner and Patty made spare ribs and mashed potatoes. Neither Patty nor I ate them; she ate a little bit of chicken and cauliflower (a very little bit; she put the food on a saucer instead of a plate, and she didn't even finish it.) I ate a salad with dried cranberries and nuts, without dressing. And we were both full. Food is beginning to be more of a chore than a meal. For both of us.

Patty hasn't been drinking enough water or eating enough protein these days, and that's why she sleeps late and feels lethargic. It seems like she cannot force down enough water unless she exercises, so she's in the basement doing the treadmill right now. She's also watching more of *The Fosters* on her iPad. I'll walk on the treadmill when she is done. Then it is bedtime.

Tuesday, January 3, 2017

Last day of winter break for the kids. It's a little difficult to separate the boys from their iPads and put them to bed. I woke up at 5 a.m. and found both boys hiding iPads under their blankets, watching YouTube. I took them away and locked them in the bathroom.

Patty did a lot of laundry today. I carried about five loads from the basement to the second floor. I did a couple of miles on the treadmill tonight; Patty skipped it today because her belly didn't feel well. She sent me to get her some wonton soup, mostly for the broth. I ate most of the wontons. The kids had pizza.

Wednesday, January 4, 2017

The kids went off to school today, and Patty had the house to herself for about six hours. She did a lot of cleaning. The house smelled like Pine-Sol and bleach. She cleaned both floors, including the bathrooms. I put away the clean dishes out of the dishwasher. I told her, "I'm doing my one percent." It's a running joke in our marriage, that she does a lot more housework than I do. Hey, at least I acknowledge it, and I try to do a little. Honest, I do.

Thursday, January 5, 2017

Patty called me today after seeing her surgeon. She is down to 294 pounds. But she is also dehydrated. The doctor upped her water intake to 100 ounces a day, and upped her protein intake to 80 to 100 grams per day. He also told her she might be lactose intolerant. So, the question is this: How is she supposed to consume 100 grams of protein each day if she cannot have any milk or cheese or yogurt? Can she just shove meat through an IV? She is at her wit's end; she even repeated today that she regrets the surgery. I never thought I would hear that. I had already figured that eating would become a chore for her. Now, it seems to be an all-day struggle to get enough nutrition for an active wife and mother of three through her much-reduced digestive tract.

It's really the height of irony. We both struggled with obesity for years. I developed the theory that losing weight *is* possible, as long as you don't do *anything* else, like work, or study, or allow any stress into your day at all. In my mind, losing weight was a full-time, all-consuming project that left no room for daily life.

Now, Patty is facing the opposite problem. She *will* lose weight. Her new, smaller stomach now makes it impossible for her to *maintain* her weight. But now she must eat tiny little bits of food almost constantly, leaving no room for anything else, like driving, or sleeping, or housework, or the kids' activities. Her desire for food has been conquered. But it's been replaced by a desire for famine. And part of me worries that might be even more dangerous for her.

Friday, January 6, 2017

I walked on the treadmill for a half-hour this afternoon; I even kicked up the speed a little bit, from 2.8 mph to 3. It doesn't sound like much, but I could notice the difference in my legs and lungs. Patty came down to do some more laundry. I asked if she is getting her protein in, and she said no. She ate about 26 grams out of the 100 she is supposed to eat, and it was about 4 p.m. I worry I'm going to come home one day and find her in a coma. She doesn't want to go to the hospital because she doesn't want to be admitted. Eat, Patty. I know it's hard, but please eat.

Saturday, January 7, 2017

Patty's birthday. She turned 47 today. She complained that is was a blah day, and I quipped, "That's what you get for having a birthday in the winter. Whose idea *was* that?" It was cold today, about 15 degrees.

We went to watch our son's basketball game this afternoon. His team won. Patty ate some grilled chicken nuggets from Chick-fil-A, and it took her all day to eat the eight nuggets. She made chocolate pudding and added protein powder, forgetting about her lactose intolerance, so now her stomach is upset. She also drank two glasses of English Breakfast Tea that she made in our coffee maker.

I weigh myself each weekend, and I was shocked to find out I gained four pounds this week. That's unacceptable. I downloaded an app today called MyFitnessPal by Under Armour. My boss, Megan, has been using it for awhile, and she swears by it. It told me I have a daily allowance of 1930 calories. So, I'm going to log my food and my exercise with this app. Patty has heard about it, but she uses the FitBit app, (and a FitBit device) instead.

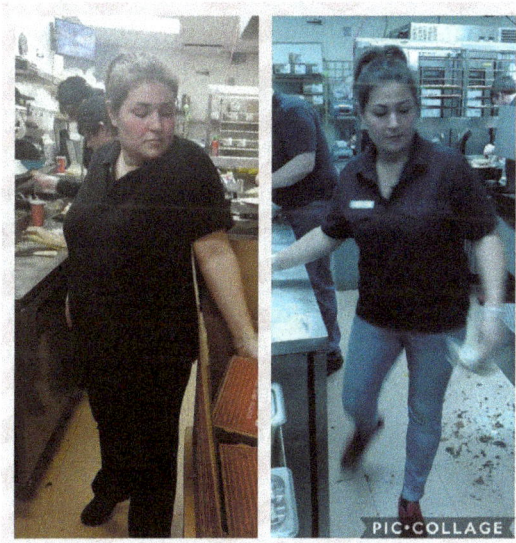

Chris's boss, Megan, who first suggested he use the MyFitnessPal app. These are photos of Megan before & after using the app for a couple of years.

Sunday, January 8, 2017

I got a big surprise this morning. Patty woke me up by climbing on top of me! She has *never* done that! As long as I've known her, she never wanted to climb on top of me because she thought she would crush me and I couldn't breathe. (That's ridiculous, but that was her excuse.) But, this morning, she rolled right on top of me and showered me with kisses and innuendo. I was overjoyed. If this is the fun, confident, affectionate woman I'm sharing the rest of my life with, then my life is complete. I need nothing else to make me happy.

Grocery shopping at Sam's Club. She is still buying some junk food for the kids, like sugary cereal, hazelnut spread, and nacho cheese chips. It's not as much as before, but I still disagree with it. We also bought lots of bottled water and pineapple and strawberries, so it wasn't all bad. Our grocery budget seems to be going a little further, because we're buying less food.

On the way there, Patty told me she is starting to get noticed by men. She said a semi-truck driver pulled up next to her the other day and smiled and winked at her. That made her uncomfortable, and she wished the light would hurry up and turn green. I told her that is going to happen more and more. She asked if I am going to get jealous. I said, "Nah, I think you'll enjoy the attention, and if it makes you feel good about yourself, then that's a good thing."

However, in the back of my mind, I got to thinking: If my wife is going to get a better offer...it's going to come from a better *me*.

Monday, January 9, 2017

I predicted before that Patty was going to lose her love of cooking, because she can no longer eat much of what she cooks.

She used to love baking. A few years ago, she sold Pampered Chef products. She also took a Wilton cake class, and still has a box of cake tools from it.

This morning, she told me she is running out of ideas for making dinner. She said she just doesn't care about making dinner anymore. Really, that's fine with me. Some people are sticklers for family meal-time, but I never have been. I'm thinking that, in the future, dinner is going to be more of a self-service affair at our house. I just need to make sure the kids clean up after themselves.

I came home today to find Patty in the living room, sitting on the...floor! I *never* see her sitting on the floor. She used to have a hard time getting herself up *off* the floor. I guess that's over now. She was sitting by the fireplace, getting warm. And she got up very easily. Twenty pounds can sure make a difference.

Tonight, Patty made a stir-fry with shrimp, peas, carrots, onions, and cauliflower. Finely shredded cauliflower that looks, cooks, and tastes like rice. We used to have to chop the cauliflower ourselves, but now it comes in a microwavable bag, which makes it so much easier. It was fabulous. I had a whole plate of it, which still came in at under 300 calories. Patty had a tiny bit of it, and still couldn't finish it all. She reported the odd sensation of trying to swallow food, but the food refusing to go down the esophagus. Drinking water did not even help. She thought she was going to throw up, but she finally got it down. But it was very uncomfortable and scary for her. She said she must have been eating too fast, and the food had nowhere to go. It was like trying to pump gasoline into a full tank...The nozzle just quits after a certain point.

Tuesday, January 10, 2017

Patty made cauliflower breadsticks today for dinner. They were very interesting, and very tasty too, covered with cheese and dipped in Ragu Sauce.

We had a productive day today. We took down our Christmas tree, and put away the Christmas decorations. We both walked on the treadmill. Patty also gave me a haircut. Our deal is, I get my haircuts for free, so that Patty can spend twice as much on her hair. It was once pointed out to me that I'm saving $11.99 on my haircut, so that she can spend $150 on her hair. But I guess I've never bothered to keep score like that. Besides, she looks pretty when her hair is done. Well, truth be told, she looks pretty *all* the time. But she *feels* pretty when her hair is done.

Wednesday, January 11, 2017

Patty is still having trouble with her energy. She slept late again today, a little bit after noon. But then she did more housework, so that took some energy. She made a doctor's appointment for tomorrow to see if there is anything else she can do. She's eating very little, but she's not losing weight as quickly as she wants, or as quickly as her doctor thinks she should. So, we will wait and see.

We had to throw away a lot of yogurt today because it had expired. I'm not eating it quickly enough, and Patty can't eat it at all anymore, so into the trash it went. I really hate throwing away food. In the past, if the kids left some cereal in their bowl, or half a Pop-Tart on their plate, Patty or I would just eat the rest. But not anymore. Food is a whole new reality for us now.

Thursday, January 12, 2017

Patty went to her family doctor today. She was complaining about being tired and not losing weight. He said she did lose 21 pounds, which was not too shabby. He said he might have to adjust the thyroid medicine she takes, because of her lower weight. And he told her it's reasonable to be depressed this time of year, because of the short hours of daylight, and a crappy weather we have been having.

Her doctor is also *my* doctor, and he said he wanted to see me also, because he hasn't seen me in nine months. That may have been fifty pounds ago, so he's in for a surprise.

Patty is off to a basketball game where Kaitlyn is cheerleading. She'll be there for over three hours, so she will need to eat and drink while she is there.

Friday, January 13, 2017

When I got home this afternoon, I found Patty napping in bed. She is still really cold and tired a lot. I was torn between wanting to climb into bed and cuddle with her, or doing the treadmill for half an hour. Ever the chivalrous husband...I did the treadmill.

She wasn't lazy the whole day. There were a few baskets of laundry that were done, and she did clean the house. But it took a lot out of her. Her suspicions about the thyroid medicine turned out to be right. Her doctor adjusted her dose to reflect her new, lower weight. She sent me to the pharmacy on my way to work to pick up the new prescription. I really hope that helps.

Saturday, January 14, 2017

Long Saturday for Patty and me, spent mostly on the bleachers. In the morning, Kaitlyn and her cheerleading squad participated in Cheer for a Cure, held at a high school across the city. We were there for a good five or six hours. Then, in the afternoon, Kyle had a basketball game at the middle school. Another hour on the bleachers. Our butts don't have the same amount of padding they used to, so our butts and backs were pretty sore when we got home.

Patty gave me a big hug before I went to work tonight. She looks really pretty with her gold hoop earrings, and I told her so. While she hugged me, she told me I was getting too skinny. I told her I still have another 32 pounds to lose. She told me I was ridiculous.

Sunday, January 15, 2017

We both slept late today. I don't know when Patty got up, but I got up at 1 p.m. I had to fix some internet problems with my sons' Xbox consoles. I did a little grocery shopping, and some work in my home office.

Patty's in the living room watching her recorded soap operas, and I'm heading downstairs to do the treadmill. But first, I have to jot down this journal entry without being seen.

Monday, January 16, 2017

I did the treadmill again tonight. About 40 minutes. These days I cue up an episode of *House of Cards* on my Android tablet and watch it on the treadmill. Each episode is good for about 40 to 50 minutes, and it helps to pass the time.

Dinner tonight was creative. Patty made...pepperoni biscuits, maybe? She took some Pillsbury dough from the can, rolled in some pepperoni slices and string cheese and then baked them. With some marinara sauce, they were very good.

For several months now, I've been avoiding eating sauces or dressings, but I made exceptions this week with the steak sauce and the marinara sauce. I eat a lot of salads, but I don't put any dressing on it. Instead, I typically put some trail mix or dried cherries and nuts on my salads. I have discovered that they are more filling that way. Therefore, I don't eat as much salad. Patty says I'm developing quite a portfolio of diet quirks, and this is one of them.

Tuesday, January 17, 2017

Last night, we put the kids to bed, and then I came into our master bathroom and took a shower. After I came out of the bathroom, Patty instructed me to close our door, and then to lock it. Her meaning was clear.

This was probably the fifth or sixth time we've had sex since her surgery in November. She told me this time was the most comfortable for her. The earlier encounters, she said, were not quite as pleasant because her belly felt full. That may have been some lingering surgery gas, or maybe a phantom fullness because her stomach was much smaller than before and she was still getting used to it. But she said she's enjoying sex more now.

It's occurred to me that each time we've had sex since her surgery, she was the one who initiated it. I have *got* to fix that. I don't want her to think I'm uninterested, because I'm certainly not!

It was a warm day for January here in Columbus. The mercury got up to the mid-sixties. But Patty still feels cold. She tries not to turn on the fireplace because she is worried about running up the natural gas bill. But she's always covered with a blanket or two when she is watching TV in the living room.

She didn't feel like cooking tonight. She sent me to get her a chicken salad from Chipotle. She ate about a third of it and had me put the rest of it into the fridge.

She was sitting on the sofa, and I laid down on the same sofa and rested my head on her lap. While we were watching the news, I entertained myself by listening to her belly gurgling, trying to digest her salad. I don't know if she could hear it. Maybe it was my own private concert.

Wednesday, January 18, 2017

I think Patty had been fibbing about doing the treadmill. She called me last evening while I was at Kyle's basketball practice. She said, "I have a major problem!"

"Uh oh, what is it?"

"The key to the treadmill is missing!"

I had to chuckle. Nicholas likes the treadmill, and I was worried he would get on it unsupervised and hurt himself. The treadmill key is a little magnet, so I hid it by attaching it to a metal plate on the ceiling above the treadmill. Even if Nicholas could find it, he couldn't easily reach it.

"Stand on the treadmill and look on the ceiling above you. You'll see the key up there."

"Why did you put it up *there*?"

I told her why, and then I said, "I put the key up there last week. I thought you've been doing the treadmill almost every day."

Silence.

"Well, I *meant* to... But I've just been, you know, too busy...doing housework, taking kids to practice and doctor appointments..."

I thought, 'and shivering on the couch under two blankets, watching *Jeopardy, Wheel of Fortune*, and *The Fosters*.' But I didn't *say* it.

"Well, I'm glad you're doing it now. I love you!"

Since I'm sounding so judgmental, I have my own confession, too. I had ice cream today. Black Cherry Chocolate Chip from Graeter's. Only two scoops, but when I logged it, it came in at 600 calories. Now I can't eat anything else until tomorrow. I'm not going to do *that* again.

Thursday, January 19, 2017

Yesterday, Patty complained to her doctor's office that her weight loss was slow and she felt constantly cold and tired, so her doctor told her to come in this morning. When she got there, the doctor was unavailable. So, she didn't see her doctor.

She is about 25 pounds down now, which I think is just fine. I don't want her to lose weight too quickly, because she'll have flabby skin and she might be more likely to put it back on because her habits will not have changed enough. 25 pounds in less than two months: she says it's too slow; I say it's a little fast. And her doctor, at least for today, wasn't around to referee.

Friday, January 20, 2017

Patty made something different for breakfast today. Egg cups! An egg, a little cheddar cheese, diced peppers and diced onions, baked in a muffin pan. I had two of them for breakfast. They were tasty.

She did a lot of house cleaning today. She called me at work and said she felt like she'd been kicked in the stomach, and that maybe she should just stop the housework and take a nap. I agreed. But when I got home, the house was neat as a pin. So, I don't think she got to take that nap.

Today, I went over my calorie budget for the first time since I've been keeping track, about two weeks. Little did I know that an individual pizza has 590 calories. I ended the day 275 calories over. So, no ice cream, and no pizza. I'm going to have to live on twigs and pinecones from now on.

Saturday, January 21, 2017

Patty is ebullient. She is excited. She is overjoyed. She lost seven pounds this week. That puts her 33 pounds down in less than two months.

As for me...well, I gained a pound. Going over my calorie budget yesterday cost me.

Our daughter took a photo of Patty, and Patty placed it side-by-side with a photo of herself from last year. Then she sent it to me. Her face is clearly more oval-shaped than before, and she has lost quite a bit of fat around her neck. Patty posted it to the bariatric-themed Facebook page she belongs to, and she received a comment, "You lost a chin!" She is still frustrated, though, with the fat that is persisting in her tummy, hips, and thighs.

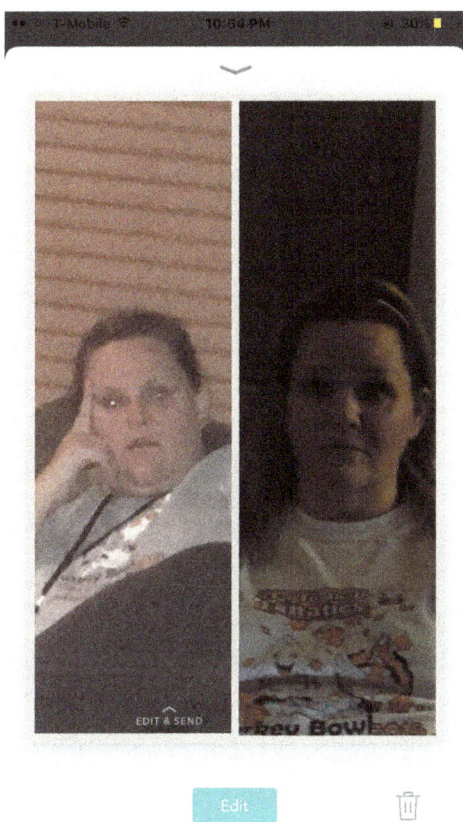

Patty lost 33 pounds, and a chin!

She fried some eggs for lunch today, and on a whim, I had her cut my fried eggs into strips and put them on my chopped salad. It was pretty good. Later, she made more fried wonton pizza rolls in the air fryer. They were good, too.

It was a warm day today, in the sixties again, so I skipped the treadmill and walked the neighborhood for 45 minutes instead. Patty didn't exercise today. I think she gets annoyed at me when I exercise and she doesn't.

Sunday, January 22, 2017

Patty has been pulling out some clothes she hasn't worn for a while. She is liking what she sees. She wore a tight black long-sleeve shirt and put a looser white T-shirt over it. That is a look she used to enjoy but hasn't worn for a while. I think she looks good. Of course, I thought she looked good before, so that doesn't really count. But seeing her smiling at herself in the mirror...now that's something special. The sun is starting to rise in her life.

I don't plan on making this a sex journal, but...two nights in a row. That's noteworthy.

Monday, January 23, 2017

The kids went to school late today because Patty took them to the dentist. Then this evening, we had high school orientation for Kaitlyn, and basketball practice for Kyle. Patty has been a stay-at-home mom since the kids were born. For the first decade or so, she was basically a prisoner in the house. Now, she is in the 'Mom's Taxi' years. She never gets to spend much time at home anymore. I work a lot, probably too much, but I'm very, very lucky to have her as a partner, to take all that responsibility off of me.

Tuesday, January 24, 2017

Patty went to the funeral of an old friend today. She was able to wear some dressy clothes that she had not been able to fit into for a while, so that made her feel pretty good. I thought she looked amazing.

She was very tired today, though. When I got home, she was napping on the couch, still dressed up. She still believes her thyroid medicine is at the wrong dosage, and she wants to see her doctor (again) to get it adjusted. She's seeing the doctor almost as often now as when she was pregnant. This is getting expensive.

Wednesday, January 25, 2017

Patty has a long evening at the school. She watched our daughter's cheerleading squad during four basketball games. Two of them went into overtime. She also was in charge of feeding the cheerleaders this time, so she brought taco supplies for all the girls.

She has to be careful when she goes to these multi-hour sports events. She needs to be drinking water essentially all the time, so she needs to keep a tall bottle with graduated lines on it, so she can measure what she is drinking.

One day, she won't have to worry about that so much. Her body will re-regulate her appetite for her new weight and body chemistry. She will be thin, and eat and drink like a thin person. And dogs who don't know me will jump into my arms and lick my face.

Sarcasm aside, that actually happened to me today. (The dog part.) I'm glad that *someone* is finding me attractive.

Thursday, January 26, 2017

Patty has been going through her old clothes, the favorite ones that she hasn't been able to fit into for the last several years. A number of them have been fitting her again, and it makes her feel really good. And I just love to see her smile.

She spent the morning running errands, taking Nicholas to the doctor, going to the grocery store and the drugstore, and hitting the drive-thru for Nicky's breakfast. That's becoming quite a treat for the kids, because we don't do it as much as we used to. And they let us know about it, trust me.

We're going to spend about six hours of our upcoming Sunday down at St. John Arena at Ohio State for Kaitlyn's annual cheerleading competition. Patty told me to think about what I should pack to eat. I'm not used to planning ahead like that. And six hours sitting on bleachers is not going to be much fun. When I was heavier, I had some natural padding to sit on. Now, I can feel my pelvic bone when I sit on a wooden or aluminum bleacher. And over time, that can get sore.

Friday, January 27, 2017

I worked very late last night, and I had to be out to work early this morning, too. After getting five hours of sleep, I got up, got dressed, and came downstairs. It had snowed overnight, so I was getting ready to warm up my van and scrape the ice and snow off of it.

I found my van in the driveway. That was unusual, because I park it on the street. Patty parks her van in the garage, because... doesn't every wife get the garage? But, there my van was, in the driveway. Running. Toasty warm. Windows clear. Ready to go.

I turned around and looked at Patty standing in the doorway. She had an impish grin. After she took the older kids to the bus stop, she started up my van and brought it into the driveway for me. Patty is my superhero.

Saturday, January 28, 2017

Patty is having mood swings. She was in a great mood yesterday, but today she is in a funk. She has a sinus infection, and she is mulling over going to urgent care to get antibiotics. She's facing a lot of laundry today. One of the washers stopped working last week, and just yesterday the heating element in one of the dryers went out. I'm going to have to get a washer and dryer soon.

Patty made me breakfast. Two eggs, with toast and jelly. She's wonderful.

She made herself a snack. A peanut butter sandwich with sliced apple. She ate about three quarters of it and couldn't eat any more. She gave the rest to me. Now, how do I log this on my app?

Sunday, January 29, 2017

Today we went to Kaitlyn's cheer competition at Ohio State. We were there for most of the day. We went to Subway for lunch; Patty ordered a chicken salad, of which she only ate about a third. I wanted a six-inch steak and cheese sub, but Patty told me to get a footlong because she had a coupon. But I knew there was no way I was going to eat the whole footlong.

So, after about twenty minutes, we sat there at our table with two-thirds of a chicken salad and half a footlong steak sub left uneaten. We were stuffed. In the past, we would each get, and eat, a footlong sub and a bag of chips, and even a cookie. Thinking of that kind of gluttony now has become cringe-worthy.

Patty managed to drink all of the water she was supposed to today. She took two bottles of water with her to the competition. However, she only ate about half the protein she is supposed to eat each day.

When we got home, Kyle ate the rest of my sub when I wasn't looking. That disappointed me; I was hoping to eat it tomorrow.

Monday, January 30, 2017

I had a long day at work today, and got home late. I had to heat up the dinner Patty made me. She made teriyaki chicken, baked potatoes, and broccoli. She was kind enough to measure it for me because she knew I would log it into MyFitnessPal.

This was another day that she was cold and tired. But those days are becoming less frequent. She did a lot of laundry today, so that might be part of it.

Tuesday, January 31, 2017

Patty's parents live across the street from us, and this morning, Patty went across to see her mom. She was coming back when I left for work, and I wolf-whistled at her. She just seemed to cut a slimmer figure, and it's exciting. She is losing fat in her face and neck, but she is still fighting belly fat, and she doesn't like the fat in her hips, thighs, and butt. However, she looks better overall, especially from a distance. And I don't often see her from a distance.

She did the treadmill today, and picked up her prescription, and went to meetings with the teachers of two of our kids. So, she has been very productive. Not a cold and tired day for her.

FEBRUARY 2017

Wednesday, February 1, 2017

*T*his morning, Patty made me a ham and egg sandwich, on high protein bread, with a couple of cantaloupe wedges on the side. I just love the way she loves me.

In the afternoon, Patty went to the eye doctor. That was a real ordeal for her. His office is downtown in the Arena District of Columbus. She had to park in a parking garage, this time on the roof. Then she had to pay for parking. And then she waited for two hours after her scheduled time before she could be seen. That's really hard on a mom with young kids who get home from school in the early afternoon.

I like doctors in the suburbs, who have parking lots, instead of doctors downtown where you can't park.

Thursday, February 2, 2017

Happy Groundhog Day. It was sunny today, but in spite of that, it has been getting colder and windier this month. I went to work with just a windbreaker, and I texted Patty and told her I missed my hooded sweatshirt. She said it was clean and hanging up in the laundry room. Then she said she'll turn on my electric blanket for me so it will be warm when I get home and go to bed. Just reading that text warmed me up.

Then she apologized in advance for not cleaning the house. Seriously? She doesn't need to clean the house every day. I hope she doesn't think I'm going to be mad about that.

She went to the middle-school basketball game this evening to watch Kaitlyn cheer. It was an exciting game, and very close at the end. She was frustrated that there was so much fouling and time-outs within the last couple of minutes. I said that's common in basketball, especially when the game is close. She said she needs to learn more about basketball so she can follow what's going on. She usually doesn't watch the game so much as she watches the cheerleaders, but the game was a nail-biter, so she really got into it this time.

I sometimes write about what Patty has eaten from day-to-day, but I was gone all day and all evening, so I didn't see what she ate, and she didn't tell me. I may have to start asking her. She doesn't know I'm writing this journal, and if I ask what she eats she might wonder why I'm so interested. She did mention she might start using the MyFitnessPal app as well, and if she does, then I can peek at her food diary that way.

Friday, February 3, 2017

This morning, I woke up and came downstairs to find Patty on the treadmill. She was watching the movie *Joyful Noise* on her iPad. She couldn't make me breakfast before I had to leave, although she said she wanted to. I didn't want to pull her off the treadmill just for that, though.

She had one of her energetic days today. She didn't complain about feeling tired, and she got a lot of laundry done. She kept our daughter home from school, and took her to the doctor. The doctor said that Kaitlyn has a sinus infection and bronchitis, so it's off to the pharmacy for Patty today.

One benefit of Patty getting up early: She has time to get all of her protein in and all of her water in. I saw a web video of how American breakfast foods are really just dessert foods in disguise. So, we try to eat protein-based foods for breakfast, like eggs, cheese, and meat, instead of carbohydrate-based foods like breads and cereals, or doughnuts, or pastries. But that doesn't mean the thought of them won't still make my mouth water.

Saturday, February 4, 2017

Well, she got to make me breakfast today. A ham and egg omelet, with toast and a touch of jelly. About 700 calories in total. It's strange that I am thinking of food in terms of calorie counting now; I used to make fun of people who did that. But, it has been having a good effect. I've lost two pounds this week. Patty has lost four pounds. So, we're both feeling accomplished.

Sunday, February 5, 2017

I ate too much today.

For the second time since using the MyFitnessPal app, I finished the day with too many calories. My budget is 1930 calories a day, but today I went over by about 127.

Patty had brought home a Southwest Chicken Salad from McDonald's, but she could only eat a little bit of it, so she offered the rest to me when I got home. I usually don't put dressing on my salad, but she already had the dressing on it. Still, I added the dried cherries and nuts that I usually put on my salads. I didn't think it would make a big difference, but it did. I logged it as 850 calories, which is way more than I want to eat in one meal. Calories can really sneak up on you, even when you're keeping track of them.

I had planned on burning off those extra calories on the treadmill, but we had to put the kids to bed first. I lay in bed with Patty, just waiting for the kids to go to sleep so they wouldn't bother her while I was in the basement on the treadmill. Of course, I drifted off, and slept soundly until the next morning.

Monday, February 6, 2017

Patty was tired most of the day, but her family just wouldn't let her rest. Her mother and her sisters kept calling her when she was trying to lie down. Finally, she gave up on her nap and put away the clean laundry that she made the kids and me carry upstairs the night before.

For dinner, she made sliced steak sandwiches, with mozzarella cheese on high protein bread. I ate two of them, for a total of 450 calories, only half the calories of last night's salad. How could that be right? And since I burned over 300 calories on a trail walk today, I still have almost 1200 calories I can eat today. I'm thinking ice cream.

Patty put a steak sandwich on her plate, but when Kyle and I left for his basketball practice, she still had about half of it on her plate, and she was ignoring it. I just know it will wind up in the trash.

Tuesday, February 7, 2017

Patty made me breakfast today. An egg and cheese sandwich on high-protein bread. This is becoming common enough that I probably don't need to journal it anymore. Maybe I'll write about my breakfast when it becomes unusual.

Today she sent me to Sam's Club to buy six cases of bottled water. She likes to drink bottled water with some sort of flavored powder mixed in it, like those little packets of Orange Crush. I like Diet Mountain Dew. (You can take the boy out of the country, but…).

For dinner, she made me a salad with lettuce, cheese and pepperoni, and cooked some pork egg rolls in the air fryer. The air fryer makes them tasty and crispy, but not oily, so that's good.

She made herself some grilled chicken with salsa and mayonnaise. She actually ate most of it this time. When she added up her protein for the day, she cheered, "Yay! I don't have to eat any more food today!"

I looked at her in stunned silence. Who on earth cheers about not having to eat anymore? Only a bariatric, apparently.

Wednesday, February 8, 2017

She told me something noteworthy today. She said she cannot eat while lying down. Further, she said she can't lie down too soon after eating. She said it makes her feel like her food is climbing back up her esophagus. So, does that mean I don't need to bring her breakfast in bed anymore?

Thursday, February 9, 2017

I got home, and everyone was in bed, the house was very clean, and smelled really nice. I know she must have done all that work herself, because the kids don't really help at all. If I was home more, I would make them help her.

She made omelettes with bacon for the kids, and I imagine for herself, as well. At least that is what she told me via text message today. When I got home, I found a pizza box in the trash. I'm thinking my mother came by and brought pizza for the kids. Patty can't eat pizza at all. I can, but I try not to. My kids, and my mom, have no problem eating pizza, because they are normal. Patty and I have become the weird ones.

Friday, February 10, 2017

Patty had a phone conversation with her dietitian today. She was told she is not getting enough calories in, and she really needs to eat more often than she does. She was told she needs to eat five times a day. Two-and-a-half months after surgery, her body just doesn't get hungry anymore. Eating is a chore for her, which is something I predicted. But she has to consume a certain number of calories each day to keep up her energy and to lose weight the right way. If she stays undernourished like she is, she'll always be fighting fatigue, and may even lose some of her hair. I'm sure that's a motivator.

She finally installed the MyFitnessPal app on her iPhone, and she friended me on it, so we can see each other's food diary. Today, she had some baby carrots, as well as an omelette with spinach. And a couple pieces of string cheese, too. She also did the treadmill for half an hour, but she needs more. She needs some different exercise, too. Her dietitian told her to do some water aerobics at the YMCA here in town. But she is such a busy mom, and I don't know where she is going to get the time.

Saturday, February 11, 2017

I did 45 minutes on the treadmill today, then I came upstairs to the bedroom to get a shower. When I walked into the room, Patty was sitting on the bed, dressed nice, hair curled, and putting on perfume. She was a vision, and she smelled awesome. That surprised me, because all we're going to do today is go to a basketball game at a middle school. She is starting to take more care in her appearance, and I think her confidence is growing. I've told her she was pretty almost every day of our marriage, and she has always blown it off. The day she agrees with me, look out!

Now that she's logging her food, I get to food-stalk her. She ate very little today, only 652 calories. An omelette for breakfast, a ham sandwich for lunch, and chicken for dinner. That's one chicken strip. And a piece of string cheese. For dinner. We are a bariatocracy.

Sunday, February 12, 2017

Patty ate a bit more today, but not by much. A total of 758 calories. She really needs to eat more, and she knows it. But she keeps complaining about how difficult it is to eat.

She gave me a haircut today. She also went to the hospital to visit her mom, who is recovering from foot surgery. She then took Kaitlyn to tumbling class. Day by day, she is whittling down her weight. And she does not seem as tired anymore.

Monday, February 13, 2017

Patty went grocery shopping today. She also bought some Valentine's Day supplies for Nicky's 3rd-grade class. She spent an hour-and-a-half cutting out hearts and attaching Tootsie Pops to each heart, so that our son can pass them out in class tomorrow. I thought, "elementary school moms are expected to do too much…"

She ate less than 700 calories today. That's nowhere near enough. For breakfast, it was bacon and egg. Which means, one egg and one slice of bacon.

The dinner she made was very good. Steamed broccoli, mashed potatoes, and gravy with lots of roast beef. I had a whole plate of it, and she had a small salad bowl full, but she only ate about half of it. Her dietitian tells her to eat five times a day. She made it to four. Is there any hope for her?

Yesterday, she reminded me that she's not allowed to have a gastric tube inserted. So, if she's in an emergency, I'm supposed to remember to tell her medical personnel that fact. That assumes that, I'm with her at that time, and I have the presence of mind to remember. We decided that she should get a medical alert bracelet instead.

Tuesday, February 14, 2017

Patty got almost all her protein in today, all of her water, and banked 823 calories. She said she ought to get up early more often and do the treadmill in the morning.

Although she didn't eat enough, her consumption has been better than the past few days. She had a one-egg omelette with ham and cheese and a banana for breakfast. Lunch was a peanut butter sandwich and a wedge of cantaloupe. Dinner was a taco salad, which was half her calories right there. I had the same taco salad, and it was great. But I ate twice as much of it as she did.

Dessert? Well, it was in the bedroom. On this Valentine's night, we tried a new position for the first time, one which our smaller bodies can now achieve.

It was fun!

Wednesday, February 15, 2017

Patty has a sore hip today. It hurts the most when she tries to bring up her foot to tie her shoe. But, that didn't stop her. In addition to the housework and laundry, she walked a half hour on the treadmill, and she rearranged the furniture in our boys' bedroom.

Our older son Kyle is notorious for hiding food wrappers, food packages, and food itself, behind dressers and under beds and inside drawers. I asked Patty if she found any food in his room when she was cleaning. She laughed. Indeed, she found a plate of turkey and potatoes under one bed. It was apparently from Thanksgiving dinner, which was some 11 weeks ago.

Kyle is not quite a teenager yet. So, I expect it's going to get even worse in the years to come.

According to her MyFitnessPal app, she is supposed to be eating 1,760 calories per day. She usually eats less than half that. Today, it was only 755. Still, she says she has not felt hungry for weeks...It's a feeling she doesn't seem to get any more.

Thursday, February 16, 2017

Patty texted me that she got a lot done today, but that she was very sore afterwards. She is going to take one of her pain pills that she was prescribed right after surgery, and she wants me to check on her when I get home. She's been very judicious with those pills. She knows they can be dangerous.

Her mother has been in a local rehab center, recovering from foot surgery. She is very lonely, and she calls Patty often. Like, twice an hour often, which is frustrating my wife. I understand. Patty spends a lot of time doing laundry because we're down to only one washer and one dryer, instead of two each. This weekend, no matter how damned busy I am, I'm going to fix that broken washer/dryer set.

Friday, February 17, 2017

The kids have a four-day weekend. No school today because of some sort of teacher training day. And Monday is Presidents' Day, so no school then, either. Of course, I don't get Presidents' Day off, and neither do most of you. If Congress decided to get rid of it, that would be fine with me.

I'd also get rid of Daylight Saving Time, but that's another topic.

Patty sent me a text telling me to get some allergy medicine for Nicholas. He picked a good day to get sick, and didn't miss school. Patty and the kids spent the evening watching movies at home.

Saturday, February 18, 2017

Patty really pigged out today. Almost 1,000 calories! Woo-hoo! She's really going through the wheat and protein bread. She told me to bring another loaf on the way home today.

I had a personal victory today. To understand just how triumphant I feel, indulge this flashback. Back in the late autumn of 1986, I was 21 years old and working at the Cedar Point amusement park on Lake Erie. The park was closed for the season, and I was part of a crew that was clearing out display fixtures from a gift shop so it could be remodeled. We were carrying the fixtures to the arcade building next door for storage. It was a large arcade, and the company stored lots of things in there for the winter, including the big Toledo scales that were used for the guess-your-weight games. Just for grins, I jumped up onto one so I could weigh myself. The scale read 204 pounds. I was shocked. I had never weighed over 200 pounds in my young life until that point.

Fast forward three decades to this morning. When I got out of bed, I stepped onto the bathroom scale, and the little display read...you guessed it...204 pounds. For the first time in thirty years, I have returned to what I call my Cedar Point weight. Back then, it was a source of disgust for me. Today, it is a source of delight.

Sunday, February 19, 2017

I promised to tackle that broken washer/dryer today, so I did. It tackled me back. Harder.

It wasn't really that bad. It turns out the washer/dryer itself was just fine. The trouble was a broken dryer outlet. The big, 240-volt electric outlet had a broken terminal that wouldn't deliver enough power to turn on the dryer. I went to the hardware store to get a new 50-amp outlet. Back at home, I turned off the breaker, removed the old, broken outlet, and wired in the new one. I turned the breaker back on, used my multimeter to test all the terminals, and they returned the right voltages. Then, I went to plug in the dryer cord, and--it wouldn't fit. One of the prongs was L-shaped, and the new 50-amp outlet I bought only had flat-blade terminals. Turned out the outlet I needed was 30-amp, not 50-amp.

It's a humbling feeling when you think you've done something so smart, only to find out that you're really dumb instead.

So, I raced back to the hardware store to get a 30-amp outlet, and was greeted with a sign that said 'Closed'. Yes, they close early on Sundays.

I had to break it to Patty that she would be without her second machine for yet another evening. I'm miserable.

Monday, February 20, 2017

Like I said, the school was closed for Presidents' Day. Fortunately, the hardware store was not. I got there as they were opening the doors. I grabbed the 30-amp outlet, and waited a few minutes for the cashier to set up her register so she could ring it up.

I brought it home, turned off the breaker, took out the 50-amp outlet I installed yesterday, and replaced it with the 30-amp one. Turned the breaker back on, tested the outlet, and plugged in the dryer. Now, both machines were humming along in harmony. I put away my tools and crashed on the couch. My family is still asleep, and I feel accomplished.

For two days in a row now, we've had spaghetti squash for dinner. Last night, it was meatballs and sauce with parmesan cheese on top of the squash, and today it was a squash bake with ground beef, onions, and cheese. I loved it. I was worried that Patty was going to lose her cooking skills, but instead she's getting creative with the low-calorie cooking. And, she's in a good mood that both her dryers are working now.

She only ate 744 calories today, still a thousand less than she should. She just can't get food down. She left a third of her squash bake on her plate when we were cleaning the kitchen. I'm glad my dinner was under 500 calories. That means I have enough left for a bowl of ice cream. (Really, it's frozen cherry yogurt. But, it's good anyway.)

Tuesday, February 21, 2017

Patty is very happy that both laundry sets are working again. She's been plowing through the backlog and now only has two loads left to do.

And she still loves to bake things, even though she can't always eat what she is baking. Kaitlyn has a cheerleading banquet this week, and Patty has been making batches of cookies to take to the banquet. She made no-bake cookies and chocolate chip bar cookies, too. She called me to ask if I was coming home early because she was out of sugar.

Even though the house smelled like fresh baked cookies when I got home, I showed some supreme discipline, and fought the temptation. I did not have one cookie. Patty made me and the kids a ham and cheese omelette instead. I'm surprised I was able to resist the cookies. Now, if she made the chocolate chip cookies in the shape of a heart, I would have been a goner.

Wednesday, February 22, 2017

Patty weighed in at 275 pounds today. That's 42 pounds down in about three months. She wants it to go faster. I'm fine with that progress. I sure wish I could lose that quickly. I feel like I have to be absolutely perfect just to lose a pound each week.

She ate 767 calories today. Still way too low.

Thursday, February 23, 2017

Maybe I've been too hard on Patty. She saw her doctor today, and she was told that she needs to drink 96 ounces of water and eat 800 calories per day. What? I thought she was supposed to eat more than twice that! According to the MyFitnessPal app, she is supposed to eat 1760 calories a day. Apparently when the app is quizzing you about your age, sex, weight, stuff like that, there is no setting that says, "I'm a bariatric, so I have no stomach anymore…"

The doctor says the water is important because it helps keep her metabolism up, so she can burn more fat. I hadn't heard that before, but, okay. Also, she was told not to drink water for a half hour after she eats. Since she has to eat little bits of food almost constantly, I don't know how she is supposed to follow this advice. It's really *hard* to be a bariatric. Some say it's the easy way out. It's really the exact opposite. If you can lose the weight without the surgery, do it.

Despite the struggle, or more accurately, because of it, she continues to lose. At the doctor's office today, she weighed in at 273. Forty-four pounds down. Many more to go.

Friday, February 24, 2017

Wow. I mean, wow. I'm looking at Patty's food diary for today, and it's just insane. She logged 1,539 calories. For weeks, I've been trying to get her to eat more than she does, and finally realized that she cannot. Today, apparently, she did anyway.

For breakfast, she had her basic ham and cheese omelette, for 230 calories. For lunch, she had a tablespoon of peanut butter. Then, it looks like she had another. And then, she apparently ate a third tablespoon of peanut butter. Each tablespoon is 100 calories. In addition to that, she had a yogurt and a granola bar. And then a second container of yogurt. A total of 555 calories for lunch. At least she logged it all for lunch. I'm not sure if she really ate it all at one time.

She made a chicken salad for dinner. It had chicken, a hard-boiled egg, a cup of chopped celery, some Miracle Whip, and whole wheat Ritz crackers. Three of them. A total of 246 calories. And for the snack category, she logged 508 calories. That's half a cup of celery (8 calories) and *five tablespoons* of peanut butter. I don't know this, but I suspect she just dipped stalks of celery into the jar of peanut butter. So, she found a way to binge after all. Well, after all her recent progress, she deserves it.

Saturday, February 25, 2017

It was weigh-in day for me. I've gotten into the habit of weighing myself on Saturday mornings when I get out of bed. Last week, I was at my Cedar Point weight of 204. At that point, I had lost weight for four weeks in a row, which is a pretty long streak. Before that, my weeks were punctuated by a plateau, or even a gain of a pound or two, before losing again. So, this morning, I was expecting that to happen.

But when I looked at the display on the scale, I couldn't believe what I was seeing. I left my glasses downstairs. That couldn't be a zero...maybe it was an eight? I had to strain my eyes. The scale read exactly 200.2 pounds. This, after a week when I was too busy at work to do the treadmill at all.

What's more, I had the courage to try on a medium-sized T-shirt. My 3XL shirts were long gone. My XXL shirts were gone. I still have a few XL shirts that I liked, but I haven't worn any of them in months. I've been wearing a large for a while now. But I tried on a medium, and it fit. It fit well. This feels really, really good.

I came downstairs and told Patty, who was in the kitchen making omelettes. She told me I was getting too skinny. She called me her "Skinny Minnie." I smiled at her and said, "Well, fatten me up then," while taking the plate of eggs and sliced bacon out of her hand.

Patty ate 772 calories today, and managed most of her water intake. Lucky for me, we both had some leftover energy at bedtime.

Sunday, February 26, 2017

I learned a new word today. "One-derland." That's when someone drops below 200 pounds so that their weight starts with the number "one." Patty sees references to it on the bariatric Facebook page she belongs to. She said that I was on the doorstep to One-derland, like Dorothy walking out of her shack into the Land of Oz. I thought of the other characters in the film, like the Scarecrow without a brain, or the Tin Man without a heart. And here was my wife, without a stomach.

After dinner, Patty was sitting on the couch. I lay down next to her and rested my head on her lap. After a while, I drifted off. While I was asleep, Patty was texting some people on her iPhone--I don't know if it was other cheer moms, or her sisters, or who it was--but each time she received a message, her phone went "ding." I started dreaming that it was *my* phone that was receiving messages, and that I was having a chat with my high-school girlfriend Charlene, who was having trouble typing hieroglyphics on her keyboard and she wanted my help. It was pretty bizarre. I would tell the dream to Patty, but I don't think she would appreciate me dreaming about another woman...

I started doing pushups today. Only 10 so far, but I'll do more later today. I'll have to get with a weightlifting coach to decide how many I should be doing each day to build up my chest and arms. My exercise philosophy is "free and convenient." I'm not going to join a gym that I'll never go to. I'm not going to buy exercise clothes that I have to change into, and out of, and wash. When I walk the neighborhood or do the treadmill, I wear my regular clothes. And I'll do pushups right here at home. I don't want any barriers to doing the exercises I need to do.

Monday, February 27, 2017

Okay, pushups hurt. They hurt a *lot*. I'm sore all over, even my legs! (Why do push-ups make your *legs* hurt?) I did thirty pushups yesterday, and another thirty today. That's 10 in the morning, 10 in the afternoon, and another 10 before bed. I'll try to keep doing them, because I know muscle tissue burns more calories than fat tissue, and I don't want to look flabby. But, really, pushups hurt.

I also did an hour on the treadmill today, after doing an hour yesterday. But, I had a naughty reason. There were some strawberry shortcake ice cream bars in the freezer, and I wanted to eat them. So, I had to burn off their calories before I let myself have them. That way, I could enjoy them more.

Patty also whipped up some banana pudding for dessert. She used Jello Sugar Free pudding mix with Fairlife high-protein 2% milk. I kept sneaking spoonfuls of the stuff during dinner, thinking it was some high-calorie container of sin that she made just for the kids. Then, when she told me what was in it, and told me it was about 30 calories for a cupful, I went "pffft" and filled a red solo cup full of the stuff, and hid out with it in my home office, like a squirrel hiding an acorn.

Tuesday, February 28, 2017

Patty is excited today. She can now wrap her finger and thumb around her wrist, and have the finger and thumb touch. She could not do this before. She tried it on my wrist, and she could encircle mine, as well. Then, she told me to try. I tried to wrap my finger and thumb around her wrist, and I was a little short. I was a little short on my own wrist, too. My fingers are shorter than Patty's. That's why I could never learn to play guitar.

MARCH 2017

Wednesday, March 1, 2017

*P*atty sent me to Chick-Fil-A because she had a coupon for a free order of chicken nuggets. She had me get the grilled chicken option for her. She didn't tell me what kind of sauce she wanted, so I called her from the drive-thru line to find out. She told me to get the regular Chick-Fil-A sauce.

She made herself a salad, heated up the nuggets and put them on the salad, and then topped it off with the container of Chick-Fil-A sauce. When she went to log it, she got very angry at herself. That tiny container of sauce was 140 calories. Much more than the light ranch dressing she usually has on her salads.

She ended the day with 844 calories, which is over her calorie budget. Of course, she was cursing that Chick-Fil-A sauce for pushing her over. I still think a calorie budget with only three digits is really absurd. But I'm not a doctor.

I've been doing 30 pushups per day, and it is not as painful now as it was the first couple of days. Before long, I'm going to have to do more each day.

Thursday, March 2, 2017

Patty has been complaining of a headache today, likely brought on by stress. She has been visiting her mom in the rehab center, and she was there for over four hours today. Her mom has not been getting along well with one of the nurses, and Patty and her dad were over there today to try to work it out. Patty told me she wished she had brought her migraine medicine. I noticed she didn't complain about her back today. Yesterday, she was asking why her back was hurting despite losing forty pounds.

She also has been feeling digestively queasy, like constipation but with an empty bowel. She took a little Milk of Magnesia, and tried to drink all her water for the day, but she went to bed still feeling it. I didn't know what to tell her. Maybe that rehab center gave her pains in the head *and* the tail.

Something positive: She wore her black velour tracksuit today. She likes that suit, and she hasn't worn it in years. She came into my home office and modeled it for me. I gave her a wolf whistle and told her, "Baby, you're rocking...2004!"

I really shouldn't make her laugh so hard. I don't want her to hurt her belly.

Friday, March 3, 2017

My apologies to Under Armour. I said a while ago that there was no setting in the MyFitnessPal app for bariatrics to customize their daily calorie budget. Actually, there is. It's in the menu under *Goals* instead of *Settings*. Patty's asleep in bed right now, so I'll tell her about it when she wakes up in the morning. Or, better yet, I'll just get on her iPhone and adjust her calorie budget myself. It just might blow her mind, how the app is getting to know her so well.

Patty complained of being really tired today, but regardless she kept Nicholas at home because of an eye infection, and she went to see her mom, like she's been doing every day. She's been putting some pressure on the nursing staff at the rehab center by advocating for her mom's care. She's not confrontational by nature, but I'm thinking this 40-pound weight loss so far might be giving her some backbone.

She had the house clean when I came home. All I had to do was take out the trash. She makes life too easy for me.

Saturday, March 4, 2017

Our neighbor, Kim, sent Patty a text today to ask if Patty wanted to go along with Kim and her dog to the local park for a walk. Patty composed a text declining, and then thought again. Before sending her reply, Patty backspaced to the beginning and accepted the park offer. She was worried about her back being sore, but she went anyway and had a great time. I hope she gets to do more of that as the weather warms up. I don't know how long she was there, because she didn't log the exercise.

Earlier today, I snuck onto her iPhone and opened MyFitnessPal. I then changed her daily calorie goal to 800. I'm still waiting for her to notice it.

Sunday, March 5, 2017

Yesterday was my weigh-in day. The good news is, this is the fifth week in a row that I have lost some weight. The bad news is that I only lost .2 pounds. The scale read a delightful-but-frustrating 200.0 pounds. One-derland will have to wait.

This morning, Patty made all of us some omelettes with diced peppers, diced onions, and cheese, with toast and gravy on the side. We went grocery shopping in the afternoon, and spent nearly $700 on this trip. Some of it was laundry soap and other non-edibles, but I'm noticing something about the food we're buying now. It not as much as far as volume, but it's more expensive than the food we used to buy. It's heavy on meat, fruits, and vegetables. A lot less cereal, and almost no snack foods, like doughnuts or cookies or potato chips. The food we're buying is also much more perishable, and while loading the refrigerator, we had to throw away some yogurt and baby carrots that we didn't get around to eating.

After the food was put away, my mom offered to take Patty to Wendy's to get dinner for the kids while I was working in my home office. Patty had chili, which she didn't finish, and she got me three chicken wraps. I came pretty close to my calorie budget, but still stayed a little bit under. I also started doing a few more pushups today.

Patty was staring at her phone while eating her chili, and I thought she might have discovered that her calorie budget had changed. Instead, she asked, "How do you log *one* french fry?"

Monday, March 6, 2017

Patty went to her endocrinologist today. She was told that, despite her impression, she's not losing weight too slowly, and that she's right on track. Her blood work was normal. She called me when she left the doctor, and told me she no longer regrets the surgery. Her voice broke a little when she told me how much she appreciated me supporting her through this.

My voice would have broken as well, if I was able to talk at all. But I was speechless.

She reminded me about how others in her family were warning her away from the surgery, citing the risks. And that I was the only one who was encouraging her, and citing the benefits. The way I remember it, I was more agnostic than that; I would have supported her regardless of her decision. But it humbled me to hear her give *me* some of the credit for her success. I only wish I was there with her, so I could hug her for an hour, or nine.

We loaded up on protein today. We had both tilapia and shrimp with broccoli and mashed potatoes on the side. I felt stuffed, and after logging the dinner, I still had over a thousand calories left in my budget. Patty only ate 684 calories on the day, but she felt stuffed too. She still managed to munch a tablespoon of peanut butter before bed.

Tuesday, March 7, 2017

Early this morning, I wanted to sneak out of bed and downstairs to the home office, so I could get a little work done, and also to write this journal entry. I did what I typically do, and listened for Patty's soft snoring so I know that she is asleep enough that I won't wake her by getting out of bed. Then it struck me--she wasn't snoring. In fact, I haven't heard her snoring for weeks now.

And because I've lost 91 pounds myself, I make much less of a commotion when I sneak out of bed.

At breakfast, she asked me, "How do you log strawberries?" Without looking, I said, "In cups or ounces, probably." I looked it up on MyFitnessPal, and I was right. I'm getting this app figured out.

Patty made me an omelette and a cup of strawberries for breakfast. While eating hers, she said with a smile, "I think I get more done in the morning now than I used to get done all day." I have to agree.

Wednesday, March 8, 2017

Patty is complaining of back pain today. Not in the lower back, but in the upper back, a burning sensation near the shoulder blades. I rubbed it, but it didn't seem to help. She doesn't know what it is or how to treat it.

She texted me tonight that she logged her peanut butter. That's how I know she is done eating for the day. I responded that I had just logged the fish sandwich and the apple slices that I ate for dinner. So, instead of "I love you's" and thumping heart emojis, this old married couple sends texts trying to one-up each other on protein. We are a curious pair.

Thursday, March 9, 2017

Patty was visiting her mom at the rehab center for three hours today, and the visit left her weary. She wanted to come home and nap before the kids got home from school, but she didn't have enough time. She's very tired each day, and she tells me she can't function without a nap during the day, even though it's rare when she gets to take one. She gets up at 6 a.m. and gets the kids ready for school; she visits her mother each day, and she helps her father by listing items he is selling onto Craigslist. I've heard of the Sandwich Generation, and Patty is squarely part of it. She takes care of her children while taking care of her parents. And she takes care of me, too, which makes it a triple-decker sandwich, maybe?

Checking her diary, I see she was on the treadmill for 35 minutes today. She is sticking well to her (miniscule) calorie goal of 800, eating 783 calories today. MyFitnessPal added today's treadmill calories to her food budget, but she didn't eat any extra. When I exercise, I usually do eat the extra calories I've earned. I guess she is tougher than I am.

Friday, March 10, 2017

Patty insists she's going to be lazy today. She was going back to bed for a nap as I was leaving this morning. Before she lay down, she had me put a lidocaine patch on her back, because it was hurting her. She blamed the back pain on the three hours she was visiting her mother yesterday. She told me through a grimace, "I don't like this...The more weight I lose, the more pain I think I have. Maybe I should just stay fat." Pain messes with the mind…

Patty logged her breakfast, but nothing else today. A 245-calorie omelette of eggs, ham, and cheddar cheese. She was really set on doing the treadmill this afternoon, but decided she was too tired, and relaxed for a while instead. Then, this evening, she took the kids to visit her sister's new house.

When I came home, Patty was standing in the living room with a glass of tea in her hand. She presented a striking impression: shiny brown hair reflecting the flame from the fireplace, a relaxed smile because I was home, and she in a thinner physique. It didn't take a close, studious look; it just took a first glance, and I could see a different woman in her more youthful, more slender figure. And I made sure to say so.

It's really awesome when a guy can win some brownie points just by telling the truth.

Saturday, March 11, 2017

We both weighed in on this Saturday morning. Patty lost two pounds this week, so she is feeling pretty good. At least mentally. Physically, her back is still sore. She had me put another lidocaine patch on her back today. After a while, she stopped complaining about her back. She made us an omelette with bacon, cheese, and spinach this morning. Now she's cleaning the kitchen and doing laundry while I'm working in the home office. She is talking about doing the treadmill today, so we'll see.

As for me? One...nine...six...point...eight...baby! Over three pounds down for the week, and I've entered that new world known as One-derland. And I'm far enough into it that even if I backslide a couple of pounds, the scale will stay under 200. Now, I'm back to what I weighed in high school, when I didn't care what I weighed. When I told Patty, she threw up her hands and said, "You're losing weight better than me, and *I* was the one who had surgery!!"

Sunday, March 12, 2017

We're up early, because we both have a bunch of work to do. Patty is making us french toast for breakfast, with sugar-free syrup and high-protein bread. We had a late lunch/early dinner, so we only had two meals today.

Also, today was the first day since, well, since I was paying attention, that I was under my sodium budget. Most of my nutrition numbers are within range, but not sodium. I've been eating way too much of it. But today, I was under my sodium budget, even though I ate pork rinds. That's baffling.

Neither of us did the treadmill, but we did get some exercise changing our daughter's bed from a full-size to a queen. That means taking a mattress and box spring down the steps, and carrying another one up the steps. I won't log it, but I'm tempted to. Patty finished the day with 730 calories, to my 1,849. No wonder she gets mad at me sometimes.

Monday, March 13, 2017

Patty really hates her arms. The skin around her triceps is loose and sagging. And she complains endlessly about it. She's been chatting with someone on her bariatric Facebook group, sharing her experience with sagging skin and vice versa. Patty has joined a water aerobics class at the local YMCA, and she'll be going to her first class today. She hopes to use the class to tone up her shrinking body. She had a hard time logging the water aerobics into the MyFitnessPal app. She settled on 60 minutes for 240 calories, which the app added to her calorie budget.

Tuesday, March 14, 2017

Patty and my mother went to Kaitlyn's choir concert at the middle school this evening. I couldn't go because I was buried with work, and I regret that. The other parents are noticing Patty's weight loss, and it makes her feel accomplished. I wish I were there to share that with her.

Wednesday, March 15, 2017

Kaitlyn's iPhone screen died yesterday, and you'd think she just lost her supply of oxygen. She declared an emergency and descended into the depths of despair. Patty, ever the resourceful mother, found an iPhone repair guy and he replaced the screen today for a very good price. Our daughter began to breathe again. I've never been a fan of Apple products, and I told her that I'd be happy to get her an Android phone. Apparently, she would rather shave her head.

Nicholas got the stomach flu and was vomiting overnight. Patty kept him home from school. She was supposed to go to her second water aerobics class today, but she was home with a sick little boy instead. She insisted she would do the treadmill today instead, but if she did, she did not log it.

Having our son home with the stomach flu worried me. What if *Patty* got the stomach flu? With her teeny-tiny little stomach? Would that be dangerous? It was an unknown, and that is what was worrying me today.

Thursday, March 16, 2017

Patty did 35 minutes on the treadmill this morning, burning 181 calories, and then she took a nap. Later, she told me that Nicky feels much better today, and she plans to send him back to school tomorrow. That's good, because then she can go to the YMCA and do her water aerobics tomorrow while the kids are in school.

She went grocery shopping again today. It seems like we're making smaller, more frequent trips to shop for groceries. Unfortunately, less-processed, perishable groceries are more expensive. The fact that a salad costs twice as much as a hamburger, and three times as much as corn chips, is a real problem.

Friday, March 17, 2017

Patty wants a new relationship with protein. She hasn't been eating enough of it lately to please her dietitian, and she worries about losing weight while keeping the flab, and about losing her hair. She told me today that she is even willing to exceed her calorie budget if it means getting enough protein. She might even stop eating peanut butter, but I don't see that happening. She is supposed to eat 80 to 100 grams of protein each day, and some days she eats less than half that.

Nicholas did not return to school today, because he was having some diarrhea yesterday. Furthermore, Kyle started feeling nauseous today, and before long he was throwing up too. So now, Patty has two sick kids at home, although Nicky seems to have mostly recovered.

Saturday, March 18, 2017

Patty kept her protein promise today, going over her calorie budget by 45 calories so she could get all her protein in. But she is really getting frustrated with eating. She doesn't want to do it. Forcing food down is an onerous, uncomfortable task that she no longer enjoys. She told me this afternoon, "I swear, if I didn't have to eat, I wouldn't."

On a positive note, I lost a pound this week.

On another positive note, Patty lost a little, too. Today she is at 264 pounds, and has lost 53 pounds since her surgery on November 29. She likes her progress.

On a third positive note, our niece Jessica visited Patty today. During their conversation, she looked at Patty and told her, "I want to have a marriage like *you* have…hashtag 'relationship goals.'"

This, from a single, 18 year old girl.

I. Can't. Even.

Sunday, March 19, 2017

Patty has mixed emotions today. She is happy about looking thinner, but she is mourning the loss of her boobs. She has gone from a C-cup to a B-cup, and she will need to buy some new clothes. Over the past couple of months, she has been wearing clothes that were abandoned in her closet that she could fit into again. But now, even *those* are becoming too big.

She has been eating more protein, which means more meat, and she told me she is getting tired of meat. Then she asked me, "What's a healthy thing to eat at a Chinese restaurant?"

"The exit sign," was my reply.

Monday, March 20, 2017

Patty finally broke our spending embargo and bought some new smaller T-shirts for me and for herself. She bought size XL for herself, and size M for me. Our neighbor Kim has a T-shirt press that she uses to press designs on a blank T-shirt, so we'll have custom-designed tees to wear this summer.

The kids are on spring break this week. Fortunately, they are old enough now to stay home alone for an hour or two, so Patty took that opportunity to go to her water aerobics class. She missed two classes last week because of our boys being sick. She really likes the class, and she hopes she doesn't have to miss any more of them.

Patty's sister Veronica visited us for dinner. She looked at me and said if I get any skinnier, I'm going to fall apart. I disagree. I still have 16 more pounds to lose before I reach my target weight.

Tuesday, March 21, 2017

Patty has been on the phone a lot today. Her mother was taken from the rehab center to the hospital because of breathing problems. They expect her to be released any day now but the mother does not want to return to the rehab center. Instead, she wants to come home. Patty and her father are trying to arrange that. That would be nice, but I also worry it will present an even greater burden on Patty. She has a hard time saying no to her mom when she feels she needs something.

Patty didn't eat very much today. She only logged 518 calories.

She nearly choked on a piece of chicken breast. She couldn't force it to go down, but she couldn't cough it up either. It's a scary feeling, and one she has complained of before. She has to eat a certain amount of protein each day, but she can't eat much at any one time because she doesn't have the room anymore.

On another note, Patty has been looking at painting ideas for the house. She wants to paint the cabinets and all the trim white. I think it's a bigger project than she thinks, but I'm keeping my mouth shut. Fortunately, I'm such a terrible painter that I know she won't ask me to help.

Wednesday, March 22, 2017

Patty went to the YMCA today for an hour of water aerobics. She enjoys it, but it really wears her out. When she gets home, she just wants to take a nap. Another thing that embarasses her, is the fact that she is the youngest person in the class. She is 47, and all the others in the class are 60 or above, or so she believes.

She only ate 670 calories today, even though she added 240 to her budget because of the water aerobics. When I talked to her tonight, she told me in frustration, "I don't like food. I wish I could just eat peanut butter all day."

Thursday, March 23, 2017

Patty ate a healthy (for a bariatric) 768 calories today.

This evening, she texted me to ask what was on an Italian sub. I told her, and she said thanks, so I figured she was going to eat one. On second thought, maybe she can't eat a sub. Was she asking for a friend? I should know better.

Friday, March 24, 2017

Our neighborhood celebrated Pi Day today. It was supposed to happen back on the 14th (3-14...Pi Day...get it?) but the weather was too cold for this kind of celebration. I wasn't there, but as I understand it, the neighborhood kids are given paper plates full of whipped cream that they throw into the faces of their friends. I'll bet it's a hoot to watch, but a pain in the Pi to clean up.

Saturday, March 25, 2017

Today is weigh-in Saturday. The scale put Patty at 260 pounds, so she has lost 57 pounds since her surgery four months ago. She still has bouts of fatigue and some back pain, but it seems to be a little less frequent.

She ate 775 calories today. One noteworthy thing is that she did not log any peanut butter tonight.

I got on the scale this morning also. I weighed in at 193 pounds, so I lost 3 pounds this week. I'm now 13 pounds away from my target. I've now lost weight for eight weeks in a row, and I have to believe I'm going to plateau again before I get down to 180. I have to be patient, and not get frustrated when that happens.

Sunday, March 26, 2017

We had a tornado warning this evening, and all five of us headed to the basement for about 20 minutes. The storm passed over us without incident, but we stayed down there as a family for a little while to watch the boys play Xbox. I'm thinking I should have a tornado kit down there; something like a storage tub with some canned food, bottled water, and a first aid kit in case the next storm targets our house, and we're stuck down there for hours or a day.

Back in the summer of 1981, a tornado wrecked my hometown of Cardington, Ohio. I was there that afternoon, and I saw firsthand the destructive power a tornado has. I've learned to respect those tornado warnings.

Monday, March 27, 2017

Patty did a lot today, but barely ate a thing. She did five loads of laundry, and cleaned and vacuumed the house. She went to the salon and got a cut and color. (She looks great, too.) She visited her mom and went to the YMCA for water aerobics. When I got home in the afternoon, she was napping on the couch with little Nicholas on the floor next to her.

Last night, I was working late in my home office, and when I was done, I decided to lower my office chair and roll it under my desk, so Patty could vacuum. I rarely do this. So I reached down under my chair and pulled up on the lever. I expected a quick drop, but instead the chair slowly lowered, inch by inch. I thought it was broken. When I rolled it under the desk, I tried the same thing with Patty's chair, which is the same model as mine. Same thing, a very slow descent.

Then it struck me. I weigh a lot less now. I can't force the chair down as quickly as I used to. Patty calls things like these, "nonscale victories."

If I keep losing weight, my office chair could double as an ejector seat.

Tuesday, March 28, 2017

Patty didn't log any exercise today, although I know she took a walk with Kim and her dog at the neighborhood park. Even so, she ate less than her 800 calories on the day.

She ate her corned beef dinner with me in my home office. She frowned at her food and told me, "I hate eating."

Wednesday, March 29, 2017

She *does* like cooking, though. She even brought me my breakfast in bed this morning, which was a happy surprise. She made me a very high-protein sandwich, with fried eggs and sausage and cheese on high-protein bread. That's half my protein goal for the day in one breakfast sandwich.

She ate a little more than her budget, consuming 817 calories for the day. But she did an hour of water aerobics at the YMCA today, so she got to add those 240 calories to her budget. So she still had a big calorie deficit for today.

After I ate my breakfast sandwich, I did some pushups before getting dressed. She watched me and told me how much I was motivating her to keep at it. "You make me stronger," she said.

Those words made me heart beam the whole day.

Thursday, March 30, 2017

Nicholas stayed home again today, complaining of a sore throat. That probably means our other kids will get it in the coming days. Before I took off for work, Patty sent me to Dollar General for some children's ibuprofen for our son, and some Crush Pineapple drink mix for herself.

She went to her dietitian today, and she brought along her food diary that she printed off from her MyFitnessPal app. That was a huge help for the dietitian. Patty was told that she's eating enough protein, but that she...get this...she needs to eat more fat and more carbs.

When she told me this on the phone, I was chortling. "Oh, you poor thing!"

"You need to eat *more fat* and *more carbs*! And it's *doctor's orders*! Oh, the *torture*!" Then I offered to bring her some chocolate frosting so she can eat it straight from the can. Aren't I thoughtful?

Friday, March 31, 2017

Patty tried some Special K Cinnamon Crunch cereal. It is supposed to be a high-protein cereal. Along with a half-cup of FairLife milk, it came to 150 calories. She also did an hour of water aerobics today. That added 240 calories to her budget today, but she didn't eat it.

This afternoon, I blew a tire on the freeway. I had to pull over and use the manual scissor jack that came with the van to remove the flat tire and install the spare. I was only a few feet from the big rigs that were speeding by. It was pretty scary. Tomorrow I'll have to go to the tire shop to see if they can fix the flat tire.

APRIL 2017

Saturday, April 1, 2017

*N*o, the tire shop *cannot* fix the flat tire. I'll have to replace it, which means I'll have to replace *two* tires. Yay for me. They have to order the tires, so I'll have to drive on the spare for a couple of days.

I was really sore today. I think changing that tire on the side of the freeway yesterday used some muscles that I don't use a lot. For example, I was doing a lot of squatting. And I was using a manual scissor jack that I had to crank. It's been about five years since I had to change a tire. I hope the next time is even longer.

We both weighed in today. Patty gained a pound, to 261 pounds, so that's 56 pounds down from surgery day. For the second week in a row, I weighed in at 193. I figured I was due to hit a plateau, and it seems I have. Last week I weighed 193.3, and this week it was 192.8, so I lost half a pound, but I still rounded it to 193.

Our 13-year-old daughter dreamed up a joke to play on Patty for April Fools Day. She was going to buy a pregnancy test, draw a positive indicator on it and tell Patty that she got pregnant. Kaitlyn told me about this plan, but I didn't think a drawn indicator would be convincing, so I texted a friend of mine, who is currently pregnant, and asked if she would give me an actual (positive) pregnancy test. Catherine came through with one.

Patty, however, was not fooled. Not one little bit. She knew what day it was, and she was ready.

She tried a recipe that her dietitian gave her. She took chickpeas and added cinnamon and Splenda to them, then cooked them in the air fryer. They were awesome! They have the look and taste of cocoa puffs, but with much more protein and fiber. She ate half a cup of them, with two pieces of string cheese for her snack. She also gave me half of cup of them, and I ate them on the way to work.

Sunday, April 2, 2017

My brother called us this morning. He congratulated Patty on the weight loss. On *my* weight loss, not hers! That left her frustrated. She's upset that her boobs are shrinking faster than her belly. She's upset that her arms are flabby. She's upset that she's sore all the time and her back still hurts. And she's *really* upset that people are noticing her husband's weight loss more than hers. I explained that she still likes to wear loose clothing, while I started wearing smaller shirts, and I now tuck them into my smaller jeans, so I guess I *am* more noticeable. That didn't make her feel better.

"I feel like you stole my thunder," she told me. "I'm going to make some French toast for breakfast. And I'm making you a whole *loaf* of it!"

Turns out, I only had four slices. But it was great. And it was filling enough that I didn't have lunch. She also made some more "homemade cocoa puffs" or cinnamon/Splenda chickpeas. And I had enough calories left over today to have a few scoops of frozen yogurt before bed. It was a good day, at least for me.

Patty walked with Kim at the park for 45 minutes. But so far, she hasn't logged any food or exercise for today. I hope she's not demoralized.

Monday, April 3, 2017

Patty did an hour of water aerobics today, and she complained once again that it makes all of her muscles hurt. As far as I know, that's what a new exercise routine is *supposed* to do. The soreness contributed to her foul mood early in the day. It is still eating at her that more people are noticing my weight loss than they are hers. That was never my intention.

What concerns me the most is that people will take the wrong narrative from this journey. In my head, I can hear people telling Patty that she cheated; that she took the easy way out of obesity. I can hear them tell her, "You didn't need surgery to lose weight. Look at Chris; he just proved it!"

But that would not be true at all. I knew that the health of my marriage required that I keep up with Patty. I was motivated by a genuine fear of losing her. The singular reason I've lost so much weight is because of the bariatric surgery. The fact that the surgery was not on *me* is irrelevant.

I did some tax work in my home office while Patty watched the Academy of Country Music Awards that she had recorded. She then came in to kiss me goodnight before she went to bed. I guess I was too engrossed in what I was doing to give her a satisfactory kiss. She told me, "Hey, turn around and kiss me, or I'm going to sit on you so you can't breathe!"

I twirled around in my chair, patted my thigh and said, "Go ahead...I'll breathe just fine!"

So she did. She sat down on my lap, and I could wrap my arms all the way around her, with plenty to spare. She said we will break the chair, and I told her not to be ridiculous. When she tried to get up, I just held her tighter, prompting her to plead for rescue from Nicholas. He tried to save Patty with a fruitless attempt at tickling me. I held her firm, kissed and nuzzled the soft skin of her neck, and breathed in the kitchen scent of taco wraps from her hair.

Amid our laughter, at that moment, my wife didn't weigh a damned thing.

Tuesday, April 4, 2017

Fortunately, Patty only skipped one day and she is back to logging again. She ate 770 calories today.

I'm looking forward to the end of tax season. I've been pestering Patty to take dancing lessons with me, which I've wanted to do for almost a year now. Although Patty seemed enthusiastic about the lessons several months ago, she always seems to have an excuse. She hasn't lost enough weight. She's too tired. She's too sore. Our son has a flag football game. I know her well enough to know it takes consistent, gentle pressure to persuade her. I'll keep working on her. I also know that once she takes her first lesson, she's going to have fun and she'll need no more convincing to continue.

She wore her 2004 velour track suit again today. She likes it, and it's even getting loose on her. Her spirits were up today, which was good to see.

Wednesday, April 5, 2017

Patty went grocery shopping today. She is still bringing in snack foods like chips, crackers, and sugary cereal for the kids. In my opinion, the kids can eat healthy, just like we do. Even more so right now, before they're old enough to make their own money and be able to go anywhere and eat whatever they want. They are still relatively captive, and their eating habits are forming now.

"I know, I know," she sighed. "But they like it."

"Priorities," I shrugged.

She made it to the YMCA today for an hour of water aerobics. Good for her. She doesn't always make it there. She is a busy mom, after all.

Thursday, April 6, 2017

No exercise for Patty today, but she ate a little more. 784 calories. No exercise for me, either, other than the pushups I do every day. I had been doing 36. Today, I started doing 45.

Patty was in a good mood today. She was wearing a pair of size 18 jeans. She had been in size 26-28 in the past. She made it a point to show off her jeans to me, with a spin and a wiggle. That made me grin. Her confident smile made me weak.

Friday, April 7, 2017

Boy, Patty busted her calorie goal today. A whopping 850 calories. And all that without any peanut butter.

Two eggs and four slices of bacon for breakfast. She made a chicken wrap for dinner, with pizza sauce and mozzarella cheese on a piece of flatbread.

For lunch, she wrapped sliced turkey around a piece of string cheese, heated it in the microwave and ate it as a roll. This is something I used to do. Fourteen grams of protein with only two grams of carbs. I haven't done that in a while, but it sure sounds good right now.

Saturday, April 8, 2017

Another weigh-in day. Patty lost two pounds this week, and is down to 259. I lost one pound, and am down to 192.

She spent some time wrapped in a blanket today. She said, "Ever since the surgery, I get cold, cold, cold!"

On another note, I noticed her scouting around the bedroom, and I asked why. "I'm thinking of getting a full length mirror, and I'm looking for somewhere to put it."

Wow. *Nothing* says confidence like a woman who wants a full length mirror. That shattering sound is Patty breaking out of her shell, piece by piece.

Sunday, April 9, 2017

Omelette Sunday, with eggs, bacon, and cheese. But, she didn't exercise today. I didn't either.

Nicholas had a flag football game this afternoon. Patty took him to the field two hours early for practice. I had some office work to do, so she left me at home and I was to meet them later for the actual game. But the game started early, and I would have missed most of it by the time I got there, so Patty just told me to stay home. That's a shame. I like watching him play.

Monday, April 10, 2017

Patty ate kind of light today, even for a bariatric. Only 576 calories. Sausage and yogurt for breakfast. Sort of a salad for lunch, with cauliflower, ham, cheese, and light ranch. We got Mcdonald's for dinner, which has gone from very common to very rare. She had a snack wrap, without the tortilla. That was her dinner. Like I said, a very light day.

Tuesday, April 11, 2017

Patty has lost another two pounds since the weekend. She's now at 257 pounds, which is a 60-pound weight loss since her November surgery. And she celebrated by not eating at all today.

I doubt that's true, but she didn't log anything. Doesn't she know I need that data to write this journal? No, of course she doesn't. I haven't *told* her about this journal yet.

Wednesday, April 12, 2017

She logged only 444 calories today. Either she is not eating enough, or she's not logging enough. I need to pester her a little bit more. She did not log any dinner, or exercise, or even peanut butter.

Patty went to the store a couple days ago to pick out some new living room furniture. It got delivered this morning. She paid the delivery guys a little extra to move the old furniture into the garage so she can sell it.

We got a new sofa, and a new loveseat. We also got...and it pains me to write this...a new recliner. A *recliner*. I proudly wrote, way back in December, that I've never owned a recliner and I never will.

And now the fool thing is sitting in my living room. I've decided that it's not mine. It's Patty's chair. I won't sit in it. One day soon, some unfortunate tragedy may befall this recliner. A broken spring, a busted handle, an ugly tear. If we get a dog, I may secretly train it to pee in the recliner. I'll say it's too big for the living room. I don't know exactly what I'm going to do...but I have sabotage on my mind.

Thursday, April 13, 2017

Today was another day that Patty overate. That's a little harsh; she logged 819 calories, which is 19 calories over her goal, but to anyone else it would be starvation level.

Her snack was the heaviest "meal" of the day, a cup of yogurt, a piece of cheese, and a spoonful of peanut butter. It doesn't sound like much, but all that snacking counted for 280 calories. It just goes to show that calories can really get away from you if you're not paying attention. That's what makes this MyFitnessPal app so enlightening. (Was that a pun?)

Patty lost another pound, so she's down to 256. It seems she's losing a pound a day now.

Friday, April 14, 2017

Our teenage daughter is home from school with strep throat. Patty hasn't really gotten sick like that since her surgery, and I'm a little scared to think about what will happen if she gets a throat infection or a stomach flu now. So, I try not to think about it.

Patty spent the day decluttering the junk drawer in the kitchen, and going through our bedroom closet, throwing away lots of clothes that we will not fit into anymore, and hopefully never will again. There is a stack of folded clothes in our bedroom almost as tall as me.

Saturday, April 15, 2017

Patty is in a turbo phase of her weight loss. She lost two pounds the last two days, down to 254, and she's dropping like a stone. I, on the other hand, am stuck on my newest weight-loss plateau. I weighed in this morning at 191.6, which I'll round to 192, same as last week. I'm actually down .2 pounds this week, but I feel like I could blow my nose and lose .2 pounds, so I'm not logging a loss this week.

Once again, Patty told me she needs to get up earlier to make sure she gets all her calories and water in for each day. It's still remarkable to think that she needs the whole day to eat 800 calories, when I could eat that much in one meal. Or, at least I used to.

I've been thinking about doing it for a while, and today I bit the bullet. I paid for the premium version of MyFitnessPal on my Android phone. Patty is still using the free version. The premium version will list my food items from highest calorie to lowest, which is a useful thing to have. It does many other things, too, which I'm sure I'll explore over the coming weeks.

Sunday, April 16, 2017

I spent much of today working in my home office, and Patty made chocolate chip pancakes for the kids. I had a lot of work to do, and I asked her if she would bring my food into the office instead of calling me out to the kitchen to eat.

That reminded me of when we were first dating, and the lasagna and cookies and pumpkin pie that Patty would routinely bring to my work for me. That seems like a lifetime ago. It's startling to think of how we both perceived food back then.

Then I thought, to hell with all this work. I went out to the kitchen, hugged and kissed her, and ate the omelette she made herself and me, right out in the kitchen with her. She really has changed my life for the better, and I'm grateful.

Monday, April 17, 2017

I haven't been on the treadmill for weeks now, because this is my busy season at work. I didn't do it today, either. But, this evening, when Patty sent me to the grocery store to get bread and ice, I took the opportunity to ride my bicycle there and back. I logged a half-hour bike ride which the app said burned 348 calories. It didn't feel like that much, though.

I'm a home-based tax preparer, and I have many clients who only see me once a year. Right now, I weigh 65 pounds less than I did last April. So, some of my favorite moments this month have been when a client rings my doorbell, and I open the door. The facial expressions are priceless.

And then, Patty will walk into the room...and the client damned near faints.

Tuesday, April 18, 2017

Patty tried a new exercise today. She went to the YMCA and took a Zumba class. Afterward, she told me it was a lot of fun and that she was sore, but happy she did it. Now, I have been trying to get her to take dancing lessons with me for weeks now, and she always has an excuse. So, why can't she take that same attitude that she has for Zumba and apply it to a couple's dance class?

Later, when she was shopping for a new FitBit, she measured her wrist to see she lost a half inch on her wrist diameter, which was another point of pride for her. She can now wear a smaller FitBit.

The hour of Zumba added 450 calories to her budget today, and she even allowed herself to eat 100 of those extra calories.

She also made a delicious banana cream pie, using pie crust, Lite Cool Whip, and sugar-free Jello banana cream pudding mix. She logged the recipe into MyFitnessPal. She thought it was low-calorie, but found out the pie crust added a lot of calories to it. She told me this after I'd already eaten three pieces. So, when I logged it, I was over my calorie budget by a whopping 318. I resolved to do the treadmill after we put the kids to bed. Then I resolved to do the treadmill after the kids were actually asleep. Then I fell asleep before the kids did.

Wednesday, April 19, 2017

We have eleven nieces and nephews, and almost all of them are young adults now, and we have speculated for the last few years about which one of them would be the first to become a parent. That wait is over. Our oldest nephew, Richard, told us today that he's going to be a dad. Now we get to speculate about which of our six nieces will get pregnant first. Just a little family intrigue.

Patty did an hour of water aerobics today, which burned 240 calories. But she didn't eat any of the excess, and stuck to 737 calories for the day.

Patty spent the day getting estimates from contractors for finishing our basement, adding doors to my home office, and a few other home improvement projects. I'm adding up dollar signs, and it's giving me a headache. Maybe we can sell the recliner?

Thursday, April 20, 2017

Yesterday, Kelly at the YMCA asked Patty if she had seen her photo in the system. It was a shocker. Patty was much heavier in the system photo. She is also much heavier in her driver's license photo.

My driver's license doesn't even *look* like me anymore. In fact, to some people, *I* don't even look like me anymore. There is a customer, someone I've seen a couple times a month for years now, who flat-out did not recognize me last week. She asked if I was new. I couldn't believe it!

Patty overate a little today, consuming 840 calories. (It still seems absurd to me that a grown adult can eat 840 calories and overeat.)

Friday, April 21, 2017

Patty underate today. Only 530 calories were logged.

Patty was cleaning our daughter's room. She was appalled by the mess, I said she shouldn't be, it's a teenage girl, they're messy. Patty insists that *she* wasn't messy as a teen. I guess I married one of *those* people!

I was in a warehouse today, and one of the guys who knows me shouted to me. "Hey, why don't you have a double cheeseburger or something?"

I yelled back, "I had my grilled chicken wraps already!"

"Uh-huh...of course!"

"With no dressing" I said with a grin. He just shook his head.

Saturday, April 22, 2017

Today was more normal, with Patty logging 725 calories. I noticed that there wasn't a lot of fiber in her diet. She has started taking MiraLax to help her bowels. "I have to force myself to poop, like, once a week, " she said. I guess when you don't eat anything, there's not much to get rid of.

She has also been complaining of allergies. We're having our basement finished, and the contractors are smokers. When they are working outside cutting drywall, or are outside on their break, they smoke. Patty can smell it as they come back into the house, and it bothers her.

I finally broke my weight-loss plateau and lost three pounds for the week. My weight is 189 pounds now. At this point, my fear when I lose that much in a week, that I will gain some back the next week. I'm nine pounds from my goal, and I can taste it. Or maybe it's the funnel cakes and chocolate covered raisins that I can taste. The cravings might be reduced, but they never totally left me. I wonder if my calorie budget will change when I reach my target weight and can focus on maintenance instead of weight loss.

I've read that maintaining your weight loss is even harder than losing the weight in the first place. How can that be true?

Patty and our daughter got new FitBits today. This week, I've been pestering our 11-year-old son Kyle to go out and mow the lawn. Today, Patty volunteered to help him mow the lawn, so she could get her steps in. She wound up mowing the whole lawn herself. She's too easy on that boy.

Our youngest son Nicholas got a cheap off-brand step counter, as well. He had over 10,000 steps today, while bouncing around playing his Xbox.

Sunday, April 23, 2017

Patty made French toast for me today. She even had half a slice herself. Then, for dinner, she had another McDonald's snack wrap without the wrap. Only 500 calories logged today.

I had told her that I still had a craving for funnel cakes, so we found an online recipe for a low-carb funnel cake. We used coconut flour to make the batter, and coconut oil to fry the dough. Then we added Splenda granulated sweetener, a dash of cinnamon, and some corn starch into a blender, and made powdered sugar out of it. The funnel cake was pretty good, but it *still* had too many calories, and I had to skip a meal today because of it.

We also spent this Sunday morning talking about...sex. She says she likes sex more, because her pelvic area feels tighter and she feels more sensation. (She is also quite a bit more self-confident.)

She also made some positive comments about my enthusiasm, my stamina, and how I don't get leg cramps anymore. Those cramps were horrible, how they used to stop the action at the wrong times. She told me she was pleased about something else, too. Rumor has it that when a man loses a great deal of weight, it has a positive--and sizeable--impact on his erections.

In our experience, those rumors are accurate.

Monday, April 24, 2017

Patty ate some more today, 813 calories. Her hip has been hurting, and she thinks it's because of the walking we did yesterday at Nicky's flag football game. She saw her doctor today and asked for a cortisone shot. It reduced the hip pain, but it gave her a headache, so I don't know which one is better.

I brought home the paint that Patty had ordered. Twenty-seven gallons of paint, plus primer. Then, of course, the painters that she hired didn't show up.

Tuesday, April 25, 2017

The drywall dust is everywhere. The contractors finishing the basement are also painting the kitchen cabinets and removing the kitchen island. Because our laundry room is covered in dust and flecks of drywall mud, we may have to take our laundry to the laundromat for a while.

Patty logged 805 calories, right on target today. She is feeling tired and sore, because she went to dance fusion class at the YMCA. I told her, "I thought it was a Zumba class."

"Oh, they call it different things, depending on who the instructor is."

"OK...so it's 'tired and sore' class."

Of course, I'm tired all the time because I work too much. (Although, this week, I'd rather go to work than stay home and do the stuff the contractors are doing.) I'm also sore all the time, because of all the pushups I'm doing. I'm now up to 48 pushups a day.

Wednesday, April 26, 2017

Another typical exercise day for Patty, in that she burned 240 calories doing water aerobics at the YMCA, but didn't eat those extra calories. She only logged 620 calories for the day.

In contrast, I ate more than 620 calories in *each* of my three meals today.

The house remodel is coming along slowly. The cabinet doors are painted white, and are spread out onto the kitchen floor to dry. The countertops are in the garage and ready to install. I guess they're still working on the basement, but I choose not to go down into the Dusty Dungeon of Drywall. I can hear a fan running down there. That's good enough for me.

Patty had the kitchen island removed, and we're going to put our dining room table into the kitchen instead. When we took everything out of the kitchen so they could paint the cabinets and replace the countertops, we piled everything onto the dining room table, which is still in the dining room. So, we can't move the table until we take everything back off of it, and we no longer have the kitchen island to put the stuff onto, either.

So, neither one of us would make a good project manager.

Thursday, April 27, 2017

Remodeling a house is *very* inconvenient. All of our kitchen is crammed into the dining room, which makes it unusable. The kitchen is all torn up, so we can't use that, either. The laundry room and the playroom are covered in drywall dust and painting supplies, so those two are off-limits. The garage is full of tools, drywall, lumber, and trash, so we can't park in it, and I can't even get to my *own* tools.

This week, I've discovered that I really enjoy going to work, and leaving the chaos for several hours a day.

Patty spent a couple hours at the home improvement store looking at backsplashes for the kitchen, and had a tough time deciding on which design to go with. She brought home a couple of samples, and asked my opinion.

Really? She's asking *me* which backsplash she should get? I thought about asking her, "Which brand of air filter should I buy for my car?"

I told her to get whichever one *she* wants. I had no preference at all. The last thing I want is to pick one, and have it installed, just so she can hate it and blame me.

Friday, April 28, 2017

We got each of our sons a year of Xbox Live Gold, which cost $60 a piece. We've debated with each other for a while about this; I feel the boys needed to earn them, while Patty wanted to give it to them as a gift. (Perhaps for herself, because when the boys are playing video games, they don't bother *her* as much...although she is pretty good about limiting their time.)

The Xbox cards we got have these 25-character codes on the back. Our oldest son entered his code without a problem, but our youngest son's Xbox did not accept his code. So, I went back to the store and bought yet another Xbox card. That one didn't work either. I got into an online chat with Microsoft, and found out his account had an expired payment method and it wouldn't accept the code until that was fixed. So, we fixed it and he was soon playing his Xbox. So, now I have an extra $60 Xbox card that I don't need. I think I'll sell it. And I think I'll throw in the damned recliner as a bonus.

Saturday, April 29, 2017

I have a new weakness, in the form of frozen chocolate yogurt. And my weight-loss plateau is back; I actually gained two pounds this week, up to 191. I blame the frozen chocolate yogurt that I supposedly bought for the kids, but that I could not stay out of. Sorry, kids, but I'm not buying frozen chocolate yogurt anymore.

Patty only logged her breakfast today. Two eggs and four slices of bacon, for 220 calories. I'm pretty sure she ate more than that, but didn't log it.

She is in a bad mood because she is discovering little dings on the new countertops that the contractors had just installed. They also got some paint on our refrigerator. She has been exhibiting a range of emotions with this remodeling project, ranging from delight to despair to frustration. I'm not going to react to every emotion, I just wish the project would get finished, so she can have her home back.

Sunday, April 30, 2017

Patty logged a full day of food today. She also made a salad, but did not eat it. That's a shame, because it was a really good salad.

She did not log her exercise today, though. I know she took a half-hour walk, because I went with her. So did our neighbor, Kim. We walked around the outside of the local high school while our son and Kim's son practiced for their flag football game. We talked about the books we're reading, and the remodeling project, and other stuff I forgot about. I got sunburned; I remember that.

After the game, we went home and Patty got a lot of laundry done, which was very inconvenient for her, because the drywall dust in the basement got on the clothes in the laundry room and a lot of stuff had to be re-washed. But, it got done, and the boys and I carried up six baskets of laundry, being careful not to touch the freshly-painted basement walls.

MAY 2017

· · · · · · · · · · · · · · ·

Monday, May 1, 2017

*P*atty's breakfast and lunch were pretty standard today. Her dinner, however, was unusual. We had broiled chicken breast, riced cauliflower with butter, and mashed cauliflower with butter and herbs. She broiled the chicken because it was too windy today to use the barbecue grill on our back deck. We had two types of cauliflower because we're trying to clear out the food in the freezer before buying more. It was a tasty dinner.

When I got home, Patty was complaining about all the drywall dust, which we thought was confined to the basement, but she forgot the furnace is down there, too, and yesterday was chilly and she had turned on the furnace, which blew a fine layer of dust all over the house. She proclaimed, "I give up! I'm not dusting this house until the contractors are finished with it!"

No delight today, just despair and frustration.

Tuesday, May 2, 2017

Patty came out of the bathroom this morning with a smile. She weighed in at 249. It was 251 two days ago. Getting below 250 is an exciting milestone for her. She is also losing a bit of fat on her arms. The water aerobics she has been doing seems to be giving her a little bit of muscle, which is helping with the so-called bat wings.

After coming out of the bathroom, she went to put her new FitBit on her wrist, and found that it did not recharge overnight like she had thought. She said, "Well, guess I can't exercise today. My FitBit is dead." That statement left me wondering if exercise only counts if you can literally count it. Despite her dead FitBit, she *did* exercise today, completing an hour of Zumba at the YMCA.

Wednesday, May 3, 2017

Today was another day at the YMCA for Patty. She did an hour of water aerobics, and even ended up on TV! A local station was at the YMCA filming a "Commit to be Fit" segment. Patty was captured in the footage of the pool. My wife is a star!

Meanwhile, a customer stopped me today, and asked, "You've got to tell me; how did you do it?"

She was talking about my weight loss, which to her seemed like it happened overnight, even though I've been at it for over a year. "What's your secret? I need to do it myself!" I told her my wife was also losing a lot of weight, and she inspired me. And I told her about the MyFitnessPal app. Thinking back, it's hard to overstate the effect that following the app has had on me since I began using it last winter. I've learned so much about food, and about macronutrients, and how they affect what happens to my body.

Patty's really not eating enough, and her weight loss is going to be uneven and will leave trouble spots if she doesn't get closer to her calorie goal. She only logged 560 calories today. Even with her bedtime spoon of peanut butter, that's not enough. Especially after doing the water aerobics.

Thursday, May 4, 2017

Patty's calorie load was not much better today. She ate a total of 650 calories, out of her goal of 800. And no exercise was logged today.

The kitchen remodel is just about finished, and Patty began moving the kitchen stuff out of the dining room and back into the kitchen. It turns out I was wrong about the dining room table. She had never planned on moving it into the new kitchen. Rather, she took some measurements and is planning to buy a *new* table for the kitchen. Each project is making me a little more poor.

Friday, May 5 2017

Patty is getting more comfortable with her body. She's still finding flaws and new bodily obsessions. She persistently complains about her so-called bat wings, and now she's stuck on the flab around her belly. She has posted about it on her bariatric Facebook group, and the women there respond that the belly is the last place she will lose fat. That's odd, because it was one of the first places I lost *my* fat, along with the face and neck area. But, I suppose men and women lose weight differently, or so I'm beginning to understand.

She has also been complaining of toe cramps. In the middle of the night a pulling sensation started at her big toes, travelled up her legs and shot her out of bed. It only got better when she walked around the bedroom.

Patty actually overate today. She logged a whopping 1,007 calories! It's rare when she overeats. I wonder what triggered it today. Maybe because she has her kitchen back?

Saturday, May 6, 2017

My wife is in a great mood. She is down to 244 pounds. When she got dressed, she layered her clothes, which is a new look for her. She is wearing a long-sleeved black T-shirt underneath a white short-sleeved shirt, and I spotted her admiring herself in the mirror, which is not something she's often done during the past 22 years. She is only two pounds away from her lowest weight of our marriage, so she says. I don't remember her being *that* thin, but I'm keeping my mouth shut about it.

I weighed myself today, as well. The two pounds I gained last week has fallen back off, and I actually lost a little more than that. The scale said 188.6, which I will round off to 189. If Patty says she's two pounds away from her lowest weight of our marriage, well, I'm already way below that. I feel like I've entered a different universe. I don't feel as if I look like 'the chubby guy who lost some weight', but rather someone who has always been thin. People around me are starting to forget the years I was heavy.

Sunday, May 7, 2017

We spent the day at Ohio Stadium watching our nephew Dylan graduate from Ohio State. The crowd surprised me; the stadium was full, except for part of the far upper deck, and Ohio Stadium is one of the largest stadiums in the country. The air was chilly but the sun was out. Patty and I were sitting in the sun, and we had to remove our jackets. Meanwhile, Patty's parents were sitting in the shaded side of the stadium, and were freezing to death.

Afterward, we all went to the Red Robin restaurant for Dylan's graduation party. This is the first time that Patty and I have been to a sit-down restaurant since her surgery. I was disappointed that their menus did not have calorie information. Fortunately, MyFitnessPal does. I was able to view the whole Red Robin menu on the app, with calorie info included.

I ordered a Simply Grilled Chicken Salad and a bowl of chicken tortilla soup. Patty went off-menu and asked for a piece of grilled chicken and a small side of broccoli. She didn't even finish it. Everyone else was wolfing down big burger platters and towers of onion rings. I was craving a milkshake, but I knew I did not have enough calories in my budget for it, so I resisted. We had the smallest check in the group.

During dinner, my sister-in-law Nina was sitting next to me, and she noticed me using the MyFitnessPal app. She asked me about it. Then she downloaded it herself, replacing the other fitness app she had been using.

Monday, May 8, 2017

I felt light-headed when I came downstairs this morning. Patty told me I needed to eat. She also told me I need to stop taking my diabetes medicine.

"I don't think you don't need it anymore. You should ask the doctor if you still need it."

That might be true. My blood sugar has been under control for a year now. I've long ago reached the point where I can keep it under control using diet and exercise alone. However, I still take the medicine, because it works as an appetite suppressant.

Patty was also right when she told me I needed to eat. She made me a bacon, egg, and cheese sandwich on the high protein bread, and added an apple that she cored and sliced up for me. You know, when you're immersed in this kind of caring, how can you be anything but grateful?

Tuesday, May 9, 2017

This morning, Patty asked me if I had noticed anything about her. That's always a terror-filled question for a husband… (Don't get it wrong!!) I looked her up and down, her hair, her clothes, and said, "Um, you're awesome?"

"I'm not wearing my ring."

She's very proud of her diamond, and it was true--her ring finger was bare.

"I took it off because it is too loose. I'm afraid it will fall off and I won't notice it."

That's a legitimate fear. Last autumn, my *own* wedding band was falling off my finger. One day, I noticed it was gone, and I had no idea where it was. Immediately, I got on Amazon and ordered a new, inexpensive replacement. But mine was just a simple gold-plated band, not a diamond like Patty's.

Patty went to the YMCA today for an hour of Zumba, where she burned 450 calories. As usual, she refused to eat those calories, and only ate 627 today. She is in a turbo-charged weight-loss phase now, losing nearly a pound a day. I wonder how she stands upright, let alone do an hour of Zumba.

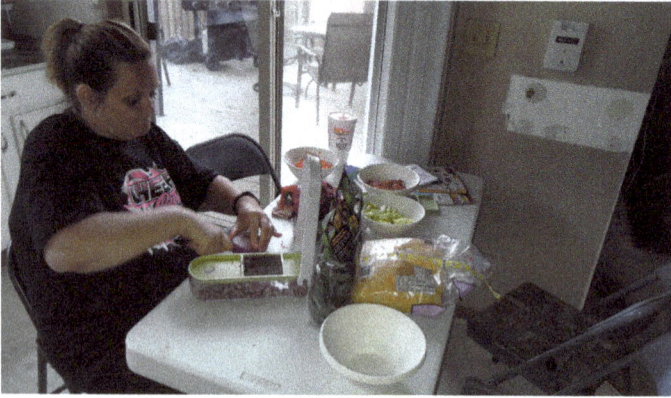

Patty making healthier food in a torn-up kitchen. May 2017.

Wednesday, May 10, 2017

Patty exercised at the YMCA again today, but a little lighter this time, doing an hour of water aerobics, which only burns 240 calories. Again, she did not eat the excess.

Yesterday, after dinner, Patty made some pudding. She took a pack of Jell-O Sugar Free Fat Free Banana Cream pudding mix and added it into a bowl with two cups of Fairlife Fat Free milk. She told me to get the electric mixer and mix it up. It was a tasty snack, and one serving was only 55 calories.

So, tonight, I wanted the same thing, but we were out of pudding mix. I stopped by the store to get some more, and I looked over the different flavors of sugar free and fat free pudding mix. Instead of banana cream, I bought cheesecake flavor. It was really tasty stuff, and easy enough for a doofus like me to make.

Thursday, May 11, 2017

Patty went dress shopping today, along with my mother and my sister. We're all going to an alumni banquet at my high school at the end of this month, the same high school my mother and my sister graduated from. My mom was even her class valedictorian! (I, on the other hand...was not.)

One of the benefits of this much weight loss is that Patty can shop for a smaller dress. She has lost *eight* dress sizes, and she has a much greater selection to choose from now. A year ago, she refused to shop for a dress at all. She sent *me* to the dollar store to find her a maxi skirt to wear to the alumni event last year. When I got there, I started a video call with her on my smartphone, and then held up each skirt in the size she wanted so she could look it over. I felt like every woman in the store was smirking at me. So, this year, I'm glad that Patty is going herself, with the other women in my family, and leaving me out of it.

I didn't come home in time to see the dress. Maybe I'll see it this weekend.

Friday, May 12, 2017

I overate a *lot* last night. When I got home, everyone was in bed, and I reverted to a bad habit I had hoped I had defeated. I found a big bag of Sun Chips in our pantry, and I took the whole bag with me to my home office and sat down at my computer with it. I began eating the chips while opening the *New York Times* website. The big story today was President Trump firing the Director of the FBI, and all the controversy it has caused. I read article after article, while munching handfuls and handfuls of chips until, before I knew it, half the bag was gone.

I've been disciplined for so long, and I thought the days of mindless eating, especially without recording everything I ate, were over. This morning, I checked my blood sugar, like I do every morning. It came in at 141, which is almost double what it usually is in the morning. Sure, I could blame Patty for bringing in the junk food, but she didn't force me to eat it. This was my *own* damned fault. Tomorrow morning, I'll have to weigh myself, and I'm very apprehensive about it.

Patty was more disciplined than me today. She only logged 607 calories on the day.

Kaitlyn texted me to tell me to buy some posterboard so she and Nicholas can make Patty a big Mother's Day card. I bought the pack, snuck it into the house tonight and slipped it under Kaitlyn's bedroom door. I'm excited to see it when she is done.

Saturday, May 13, 2017

I had been getting very little sleep this week, and today was my day to make up for it. I slept in until noon, and only got up because Patty brought my breakfast up to me. What a treat! She made me some fried eggs and Canadian bacon, along with some toast with jelly and margarine. Before she let me eat it, she sent me into the bathroom to weigh myself.

Because of my total lack of discipline with the Sun Chips yesterday, I managed to gain a pound this week. I went from 188.6 to 189.6, according to the scale. I decided to leave my weight at 189 when logging it into MyFitnessPal. I also did my 16 pushups before I ate.

Patty also weighed herself this morning. After losing six pounds last week, she was disappointed this week because she only lost .2 pounds. She says that it's unfair, because the surgery should guarantee a big weight loss every week. She's getting impatient. Then she blamed the peanut butter that she has been eating each day, and told me she may swear off peanut butter so she can get on track again.

That was a big statement.

This afternoon, we both went to Home Depot to get soil, rocks, and plants for our backyard vegetable garden. We got some cherry tomato, cucumber, and zucchini seeds for planting. We also got a few five-gallon buckets. We're going to fill the buckets with garden soil and then plant the zucchini in them to see if they will grow in the buckets. In the past, we've had the zucchini in the garden just kind of take over and crowd out the other plants in the garden, so this year we're going to separate the zucchini from the other plants to see if that makes a difference.

On the way home tonight, I stopped and bought some Mother's Day flowers for both Patty and my mom.

Sunday, May 14, 2017

Today was another flag football game day for our son, and his team actually won. That's the first time this year. The victory was exciting for the boys and for the moms on this Mother's Day.

Patty, our neighbor Kim, and I took a walk around the high school campus while the boys were practicing before the game. The walk took about 20 to 30 minutes, but it was at a slow pace in the wind, so we did not log it.

The walk and the game was a nice respite from the chaos that is going on in our house. The first attempt at our kitchen remodel didn't go as well as Patty liked, so she called the contractor back out to make repairs. Cooking is very difficult with the kitchen torn up, so we had McDonald's for dinner. Patty had a grilled chicken snack wrap, without the tortilla. I snuck a handful of the kids' french fries, and I felt at least guilty enough to log them. I also had a Southwest grilled chicken salad, and I took Patty's discarded tortilla, tore it into strips, and added it to my salad. It was pretty tasty that way. We are a symbiotic pair of dieters.

In a twist of irony, I learned that I have some food-stalkers of my own. My sisters-in-law Tiffany and Nina have been looking at my food diary that I share on MyFitnessPal and they've been commenting to Patty about my food choices. I don't know if I'm supposed to feel self-conscious about that, but I don't.

For a couple of hours tonight, Patty and I prepared the living room for the painter, whose name is Nancy. We removed the outlet covers and switch plates, and took down the flat-screen TV and the mounting bracket. I also took the blinds down from the windows. Remodeling sucks.

Monday, May 15, 2017

Nancy arrived right on time and began painting the living room. I was gone most of the day, and came home in the afternoon as she was getting close to finishing. The room looked very nice, and had that fresh paint smell. Patty was trying to stay out of her way, so she went upstairs to tidy up. When I got home, I found her napping in bed, along with Nicholas. That looked like a good excuse to take a rare nap myself, so I shoved the boy over toward his mom and climbed into bed with them. We napped for about an hour, until Nancy was finished for the day.

It was tempting to bring in some more take-out for dinner, but Patty forced herself to cook. She made us some pan-fried chicken with mashed potatoes and broccoli. We ate out on the back deck, because it was so nice today.

While we were eating, Patty's mom called me to her house across the street so I could help her turn on her air conditioner. And that was another change that I have noticed since my weight loss.

When I was heavier, air conditioning used to be my friend, my crutch, my narcotic. I would turn it on in March or April and use it until October or November. If the air conditioner failed in my car, I would *rent* a car just so I would not have to suffer in the humid Ohio heat. Our home has central air, but I still used a portable air conditioner in our bedroom so we could sleep more comfortably.

Then, last summer, as I passed 250 pounds on my way to about 220, I noticed that I could handle the heat better. I even stopped using the air conditioner in my car, because I noticed that the cooler I was, the hungrier I got. Today, in the middle of May, I have yet to use the car's air conditioner, because I'm much more comfortable now. We haven't even used it in our *house* yet.

Another thing: I had to use our eight-foot ladder a few times during this remodel. The ladder comes with a weight limit of 225 pounds, which made me nervous when I was heavier. But now I'm only 189, and I don't worry about that anymore.

Patty calls these 'non-scale victories'. They're coming in bunches now.

Tuesday, May 16, 2017

Patty had a honey-do list for me this evening. The job I was to tackle first was the easy one: replacing the kitchen outlets with ones that match the new kitchen decor. There were about six outlets to replace, and I figured it would take maybe an hour to do.

Five hours later, I finally got the last outlet to actually work.

Nothing was going right. I would get one working, then the one I did before that would stop. Or, my tester would indicate the wires were reversed. Even though I was careful to turn off the breaker after each test, I *still* managed to shock myself. Twice. I was so frustrated that I cracked open the gallon of frozen chocolate yogurt we had, and I wound up eating the entire gallon. I overate by more than 1,400 calories, and I just didn't care.

I don't think Patty cared about logging today, either, because she didn't log at all. I'm guessing she was just as frustrated that I wasn't getting my project list done.

Wednesday, May 17, 2017

The remodeling blues continue. A big bucket of our paint is missing, and we think the contractor walked out with it. So, we can't finish painting. This work is much more disruptive to our routine than we had expected, and our weight-loss strategies are suffering.

Patty stayed within her calorie goal, and I applaud her for that. She logged only 620 calories today. But yesterday and today, I blew *my* calorie budget to smithereens. I spread the logging of the frozen yogurt over two days, so it wouldn't look as bad, but I'm going to dread the scale this Saturday. This house project has left both of us exasperated and drained, and we really need to take this much slower. I can barely write this journal.

Thursday, May 18, 2017

Today things went from bad to worse. We needed to move our bedroom furniture into the center of our bedroom for the painters. As we were moving our bed, the center supports got ripped out of the frame, so now we can't sleep on our bed. It seems when you remodel, you not only need a crew to do the painting, but you need another crew to do the preparation work and the repair work for all the stuff you break.

Patty logged 690 calories today, so she is staying disciplined amid the chaos. I managed to stay within my budget as well, logging 1,770 calories out of my 1,930 per day. That was probably because I stayed away from the house all day and evening while I was at work.

Afterward, I did manage to (somewhat) fix the bed supports so we could at least sleep in the bed tonight. And I also got the living room TV hung back on the wall. This was the project

I was supposed to do a couple of days ago, and couldn't because the kitchen outlets took all my time. So now, Patty can watch her TV again. Her mood is considerably brighter now.

Friday, May 19, 2017

There is a proverb that goes along with remodeling: "That which will get moved, is that which will get broken."

We moved the home office furniture away from the wall, and it was a little precarious. Precarious enough that when Nicholas went to retrieve something from Patty's desk, he managed to knock the whole desk over, with her computer, monitor, and printer along with it. Before I went to work, I had to move all that debris away from the wall so the wall could be painted, and I didn't have time to bother seeing what was broken and what was not. So, I left for work in a crappy mood. Living here sucks right now, and I'm glad I can get away.

I overate today, but just a little bit. I went over my budget by 60 calories. Patty didn't log anything at all, so I can't tell whether she is more relieved that the TV is back up, or more frustrated that her computer may be broken.

Saturday, May 20, 2017

This is the day I've been dreading. After overeating much of this week, it is judgement day. I got up, went into the bathroom and stepped on the scale.

Before I disclose the reading, I'll share a bit of philosophy. The scale, I've learned, is a most fickle beast. Attempts to please it is often counterproductive; conversely, treating it with apathy will sometimes get its attention.

That being said...I lost two pounds this week. I'm at 187.

Patty weighed in at 243, a loss of only .2 pounds for the week. She is disappointed.

"You're going to leave me because of my ugly arms!" she cried.

On the flip side, some of the rooms in the house are painted and we can move the furniture back into place. So, I won't be able to leave her for some young supermodel until I put this house back together.

Sunday, May 21, 2017

Before we got out of bed this morning, Patty was in a good mood.

"Guess what?" Running her fingers up and down the sides of her chest, she said, "I can actually feel my ribs!"

She invited me to reach over to feel them for myself. They were round, soft, and delightful.

"Those *aren't* my ribs…"

There was no flag football today because of a forecast of thunderstorms all day. That's bad, because the make-up game will be next Sunday, during the Memorial Day weekend, and we're not sure all of the team will show up. We might have to forfeit our game if we can't field a team. It's also good, because it gives us an opportunity to put some of the house back together after two weeks of interior painting. That should put us both in a good mood.

Patty made something new for dinner tonight. It was lasagna, without the noodles. Lean ground beef, cottage cheese, and mushroom pasta sauce, served in a bowl. We ate it alongside the salads Patty had stored in mason jars last week. Even though it was very tasty, we called it 'slop'.

Monday, May 22, 2017

The painters are done with the first floor, and today they start the kids' bedrooms upstairs. They'd better get a move on, because this is the last week of school, and I hope their rooms are put back together before they are home full-time.

Patty logged 650 calories today. A ham and cheese omelette for breakfast, and only some cookies-and-cream greek yogurt for lunch. She loves that stuff, and only one grocery store in our area sells it, so she likes to stock up when she is on that side of town.

She was talking to her family on the phone, and they mentioned having a cookout for Memorial Day. That was something we used to do every year, but no more. I heard Patty say, "It costs money, and I don't enjoy it anymore."

From now on, our summer holidays will involve family outings and new experiences, instead of the same old cookouts and fly-ridden potato salad. I'm looking forward to that. This weekend, though, we'll go to that make-up flag football game and do some more remodeling.

She went to her family doctor today, and she had lost another pound in the last two days, weighing in at 242. She was also happy that she could use the regular sized blood pressure cuff instead of the larger one. She also showed the doctor a photo of me, and she told me that he said I could stop losing weight now. Gee, thanks, doc. But I still have another seven pounds to go.

Tuesday, May 23, 2017

So, when I got home today, Nicholas was sitting on the floor in the corner playing with his iPad. Patty asked him if he was eating anything, and he said no. Then she asked me to check. I walked over to him, and noticed he had hidden a cup of yogurt under the entertainment center.

Now, we don't mind him eating yogurt, but we mind him lying about it, and hiding his trash under the furniture, which is out of character for him. (It's something his older brother would do.) I wanted to stand him in the corner for nine minutes (he's nine years old). Patty shook her head no, and told him if he does it again, he's in the corner. I think she's too lenient.

Back on March 26, I wrote about the local tornado warning sirens sending our family of five to the basement for a while. Tonight, Patty was cleaning out Nicky's school backpack and she found a story he had written about the tornado warning. He thought it was very cool that we allowed him to eat snacks down there that day, because we usually don't.

Maybe he will write a neat journal one day.

Wednesday, May 24, 2017

"It's so bad when you have to *force* yourself to eat," I overheard her saying today. She really does struggle with that. She does a lot of planning, whether she follows it or not. On a positive note, she's happy that she can feel, and see, her collarbone. And her ribs. She has a skeleton after all. Who'd have thunk it?

Thursday, May 25, 2017

She's at 242 still… and mad she is not losing. She wants to look up her food diary to see what she was eating the week she lost six pounds.

While I was brushing my teeth this morning, Patty came into the bathroom and stood next to me, looking at the both of us in the mirror. She smiled and said she looks young. She's wearing size 16 jeans today, and she thinks they look great on her. She used to wear size 24.

When we came downstairs, she went down ahead of me, and she bounced down the stairs like a teenager. I remember the days when she would hold tight to the railing and groan with pain with each step. Now, there seems to be no stopping her.

Friday, May 26, 2017

Today was the last day of school for the kids. Kaitlyn was leaving the eighth grade, and thus it was her final day at her middle school. The parents gathered at the school to give the kids a "clap out," where the parents line up along the walls and applaud the kids as they parade through the halls for the last time. I made it to the school to participate, but I was behind the crowd, and Kaitlyn didn't see me. I'm not as big a target as I used to be.

Later today, I was putting some stuff away in storage, and ran across our wedding album. We were both close to 300 pounds each on our wedding day 17 years ago. I plucked out a few photos to show them to Patty. The difference was astounding, and I feel very close to her today.

Later, the son of a co-worker dropped by to pick up his dad from work. This boy hadn't seen me in a few years, and didn't recognize me right away. When I said hi to him, he gaped at me, and even used some profanity, but in a good way.

Saturday, May 27, 2017

Another weigh-in Saturday. We each lost a pound, Patty is at 241 and I am at 186. That puts us in a good mood for our big event tonight, the alumni dinner and dance at my small-town high school.

We had some french toast again for breakfast, and we like it with the zero-calorie powdered sugar that Patty makes in a blender with Splenda and cornstarch. The breakfast was late, so we skipped lunch, and we'll eat some chicken and potatoes at the alumni dinner.

She had thought about getting her hair done for tonight, but decided to do it herself. This afternoon, she asked me to make her a cup of tea, and to bring it upstairs to her. When I did so, she asked me to hand her the curling iron out of the bathroom. I reached under the counter to grab it, and handed it to her.

"No, I need the green one."

I reached further under the counter and fetched another one.

"No...the *green* one!"

How many curling irons does one woman need?

I found the green one and handed it to her. Then she asked for the blow dryer.

"Which one?", I replied. Her look said, "I only have one, stupid."

Some days, I accept my own bald head as a blessing.

The alumni dinner was fun, as my mother, sister, brother, and their spouses had dressed up in gowns, black ties and tails. We got lots of pictures and lots of comments. On the way home, Patty was craving some protein, but we were in a rural area where there were not many places to eat after dark. We did find an out-of-the-way Arby's and Patty got a junior roast beef sandwich and ate it without the bun. I looked at MyFitnessPal and noticed that she logged it for lunch today, even though she ate it close to midnight.

Sunday, May 28, 2017

On the morning after the event, my family gathered for breakfast at Bob Evans. Patty and I both had a western omelette made with egg whites, and a side of cantaloupe.

My brother seemed really impressed with our weight loss, especially mine, which was striking to me; he's my older brother, and I don't think I've ever been able to impress him at all. He summed up my strategy by saying, "This is what happens when you listen to your wife." *His* wife agreed.

Later, Patty and I went to see Nicholas play that flag football game that got postponed last week. I was worried that we wouldn't have enough players and would have to forfeit, but that didn't happen to us. It actually happened to the *other* team. Even though they had to forfeit, we all wanted to play anyway, so our team loaned them a couple of players in rotation so the kids could all play football. I thought that was really cool.

After the game, I carried our chairs to the van, while Patty stayed behind to chat with the other moms. (The kids and I call her "Chatty Patty.")

Moments later, out of the corner of my eye, I noticed an attractive football mom walking from the field toward the parking lot. I took a double take, and then I saw that this hot mom was...*Patty*! I don't see her from a distance that much, and today, at first glance, she didn't appear to be the woman I'm married to. She appeared to be the type of woman my wife would slap me for looking at.

Tonight, Kaitlyn had her first 'paid' babysitting job, watching two young kids in our neighborhood. She came back home with the money the parents paid her, and she was all smiles.

It was a pretty good day.

Monday, May 29, 2017

Patty only logged her breakfast today. I know she ate more than just breakfast, because we managed to host a Memorial Day cookout anyway, mostly by default. We really didn't make any other plans, and Patty's family migrated to our house to see our new paint and look over the remodeling. There were frosted cookies, and apple pie, too. But they were store-bought, and not homemade. My kids ate the cookies, and I had one slice of apple pie, but Patty was very disciplined. She only ate small amounts of meat and fruit, but she didn't log it for some reason. She also tried something new: she made some sugar free pudding and filled some freeze-pop molds with it to make frozen pudding pops. Delicious!

Tuesday, May 30, 2017

I was disappointed this morning when I went into my home office and found my desktop computer wouldn't turn on. I had to run to work, so I couldn't even troubleshoot what was wrong. It's an unnerving feeling when that happens. I felt disconnected all day.

When I got home, I tried another power cord on the computer, and that didn't work. So, I figured the problem was in the power supply. I had another similar desktop gathering dust in the basement, so I pulled the power supply from it and transferred it to my office desktop. It worked. And it was much quieter, as well. But, this computer is getting a few years old now, and I've really been thinking of getting a laptop.

Later, Patty was in the laundry room while I was cleaning the crawl space. I was grumbling about all the clutter up there, and how we needed to get rid of some of it. She told me to stop with the attitude.

"Well, come up here and cheer me up, then!"

"In the crawl space?"

"Sure! In fact, this is one room where we haven't...umm... you know…"

"Pffft….you're stupid!" She went back to folding towels, and I went back to declutter and dust.

We made more "slop" or lasagna without noodles. Very high in protein, and very tasty, too.

After dinner, Patty used the freeze-pop molds that we made frozen pudding pops in, and used them to make frozen yogurt pops. We did cookies-and-cream yogurt and cherry yogurt. We let them freeze overnight.

Wednesday, May 31, 2017

Patty weighed herself this morning. She has lost another couple of pounds, so she's down to 239 now. That put her in a good mood before going to the doctor to give blood.

Despite feeling good about her weight loss, she hates the bat wings under her arms. She mentioned plastic surgery to remove them. Patty was discouraged, though, because she knew such skin removal surgery would be expensive.

While she was on the phone talking to her sister about the skin surgery, I dropped to the bedroom floor and did my 16 pushups. Then I crawled into the bed next to her, pointed to my own triceps, and whispered, "Pushups are free."

JUNE 2017

Thursday, June 1, 2017

Speaking of pushups, I'm trying a new strategy starting this month. I've increased my sets to 20 pushups three times a day, but I'm only doing them every other day. Therefore, I'm giving my muscles a rest every other day. I don't know what effect that will have, but I've read on the internet that it's good to do that. And hey, the internet is never wrong, is it?

Patty got *her* exercise in by tearing up the linoleum from the kitchen floor. We're having a new laminate floor laid soon, and Patty decided to start the preparation work by removing the existing floor and the thin subflooring, too. What a mess!

Friday, June 2, 2017

Amazon delivered Patty a set of little hand weights today. I believe she plans to use them to tone up her arms and reduce the bat wing problem. How effective that will be, I have no idea.

It was a little slow at work today, and I was in the library writing this journal. But I had to stop, because my left eye was stinging and watering and feeling awful. It was bad enough I stopped into a local Urgent Care to have it checked out. When they asked me to step on the scale, it registered 196 pounds. Of course, I was wearing clothes and shoes, and carrying my keys, cell phone, and laptop. When I weigh myself at home, I'm naked, so that 10 pound difference wasn't too alarming, but still.

The doctor checked for debris in my eye and looked for any scratches on the cornea. He found none, so he proclaimed it an allergic reaction and told me to take some Allegra. I'm not sure that was worth the co-pay.

Saturday, June 3, 2017

Well, I *thought* I was at 186. Today was weigh-in day for us, and I gained this week. The scale oscillated between 188 and 190. That was disappointing, but I decided to log it as 190, hoping to have a nice drop next Saturday. Patty had a losing week, though. She's down to 237, which is an 80 pound weight loss in about six months. I'm really proud of her.

This morning, she was making an omelette for our son, and I was emptying the dishwasher, when she turned around to face me, and threw her arms wide for a hug I hugged her tightly and kissed her cheek and refused to let her go. After a bit, she said, "Let me go! My butter is melting!"

"Your fat is melting, too," I replied.

Sunday, June 4, 2017

Yesterday afternoon, we drove a couple hours from Columbus to Cincinnati so Nicholas could play in his flag football tournament at University of Cincinnati's Nippert Stadium. We stayed over Saturday night in a hotel, and at this hotel each adult guest is given coupons for three free alcoholic drinks. Patty didn't drink, but I decided to go ahead and partake. I had three tequila sunrises (or, tequilas sunrise?). The six-ounce cups were about half full of ice, so I figured I drank about nine ounces of the stuff. When I logged it into MyFitnessPal, I was disappointed to see I drank over 300 calories, busting my calorie budget by 250. It's a good thing we only stayed one night.

We ate breakfast at the hotel this morning. Patty had eggs, ham, cheese, and salsa for a 203-calorie breakfast. We ate lunch at the stadium, and she packed a blueberry yogurt and some sliced turkey for lunch. She didn't log a dinner, since we were on the road returning to Columbus. For a snack, she had most of a bag of protein chips and some peanut butter. A total of 573 calories.

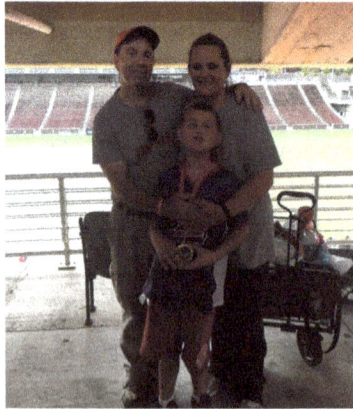

Like   Comment   Send

Charlene and 41 others

Stacey
You guys are melting away!! So skinny!!

Like   Reply   2

Megan Agreed!!!

Patricia You guys are so funny!...

I stayed under my calorie budget today, but just barely. I had a big breakfast at the hotel, and a salad at Panera Bread for lunch. I had to use my app to see what the calorie count was for the items at Panera, since the menu board had no calorie information. MyFitnessPal is a very handy app to have.

Monday, June 5, 2017

This was the second day in a row Patty ate less than 600 calories. That's not good for her, especially because she is getting the floor ready for new laminate, work that burns a lot of calories.

We ordered new blinds online, and they arrived the other day. I started to hang them, but when Patty saw them, she exclaimed that they were not wide enough. That's because when I measured the windows, I measured inside the trim instead of the outside, so we ordered the blinds half an inch short. That's 14 sets of blinds. I think they look okay, but she's not very happy at all right now. I have failed her once again.

Tuesday, June 6, 2017

Patty didn't log anything at all today. She has been complaining of stomach cramps, and general soreness from all the work she's been doing. Also, maybe she is sick because I botched the blinds. I don't remember seeing her eat anything today, but I wasn't home until the evening.

I do remember her exclaiming, "I feel so stuffed...like I swallowed a watermelon!"

Wednesday, June 7, 2017

This was the second day in a row that Patty didn't log any food into MyFitnessPal. I really hope she is not abandoning it. She's been doing so well!

We have had this new furniture for a couple of months now. Patty liked it because it was made of this faux-leather material that was easy to clean. But now, she is complaining that it is not very comfortable to sit on. She actually called me today and told me she was thinking about selling it.

Ordinarily, I would throw up my hands at something like this. But, it's an attractive idea for a couple of reasons: One, it would be nice to be rid of the furniture while the new flooring is laid, and two, what better way to get rid of that evil recliner?

Thursday, June 8, 2017

Patty is back to logging her food. She got up a little above 600 calories today, but not by much. A total of 638 calories. Is her stomach still bothering her? Or is it her back? Either one would make her not want to eat.

We thought summer might be a break, but Patty is incredibly busy, each and every day. All three kids have some sort of summer activity to be driven to and from, and Patty called me today exhausted and dying to have just a little bit of a break.

She really is the pillar that holds this family upright. I deeply appreciate her, and I think I'm going to get her flowers tonight, just because.

Friday, June 9, 2017

Earlier this week Patty laid down mulch around the house, and soon after she got a bad rash on her face and neck. The urgent care doctor prescribed steroids, and the steroids are making it hard for her to lose weight because she said she's retaining water. It's always something.

Patty also had a garage sale this morning. She only had one customer stop by, and buy $8 worth of used clothes. That's it. I think it's too late in the year for a garage sale. It's going to be hard to declutter this house.

I *did* get her the flowers, and a card, too. She said the card made her cry. Score for me!

Saturday, June 10, 2017

Another weigh-in Saturday for Patty and me. Patty is frustrated; she did not lose any weight this week. She says the steroids make her want to drink lots of water, but it hurts her belly to drink it too quickly. I had a fair drop of 3.2 pounds, tipping the scale at 186.8, which I will log as 187 into MyFitnessPal.

Even though we both have so much to do this weekend, we both wasted time by cuddling in bed this morning. Patty was lamenting all the stuff she needed to do, but I guess I was making her too comfy to get out of bed.

Our kitchen is not very useable with the floor torn up, so Patty made French toast on the barbecue grill on our back deck. It was a little different, but good nonetheless. Patty ate very little herself today. I know she drinks a lot of water, though, and she uses some sugar-free apple mix in her bottled water.

My nephew Jonathan walked into the house today to pick up his sister, Jaclyn, who was staying the night with our daughter. He hasn't seen me in months, and he yelled, "OH MY GOD!!!" when he saw me in the kitchen. I just shrugged and smiled. Later, Patty was doing laundry and I was up in the crawl space cleaning it out.

Patty said, "I thought after 80 pounds lost, I would get some of those 'OMG' moments myself, but I guess not!" I told her, "You need to get some smaller clothes."

Patty and her sister Tiffany started tearing up more of the floor today. I feel she's charging into this flooring project before doing the proper planning, which will lead to disruption and chaos. I'm furiously setting up my new laptop because I know my office will be torn up for a while. And if I don't keep up on this journal every day, I'm going to forget these little anecdotes that make up the story of this transformation we're going through.

Sunday, June 11, 2017

Lots of floor work today… Lots!

We've been pulling up more of the floor today, this time in the living room, dining room, and home office. Our driveway is full of old carpet, padding, tack strips, and other trash that we will have to dispose of. Patty said her sister will put it in her truck and take it to the dump, but her sister is doing the same project at *her* house and I can't imagine she is going to have the energy.

Remodeling is really disruptive if you're doing it in a house where, you know, people have to live.

Monday, June 12, 2017

We had to take a little break. We still have to pull nails and staples out of the floor before laying the new laminate, but neither of us want to do anything. When I got home today, Patty and I cuddled on the couch for maybe three hours. I even took a nap. She said she really bit off more than she could chew. I knew she was talking about the floor, but...that's not a very funny joke for a bariatric, I thought.

I stayed up late to do a little writing, and I poked around in the freezer for something to eat. I found some riced cauliflower and sweet potato mix, and heated it up and ate it. With some butter, it was very good. And only 200 calories for the whole bag.

Tuesday, June 13, 2017

This morning, Patty said, "I'm only 19 pounds down from my last doctor's appointment, and I need to be 25 down...I'm so frustrated! My doctor is going to hate me!" She is blaming the steroid treatment for making her hungry and thirsty. She says she has been at 237 for weeks now. I'll have to go back and see if that's true. I think she's doing fine.

And wouldn't you know it... Patty was only a half-hour into her workout today, when our son's football practice was cancelled and Patty was called away to pick him and his friends up because there was lightning. She wound up taking *four* boys to their homes because their moms couldn't come pick them up. My poor wife just can't get a break.

We've been preparing the main floor of our home for new laminate flooring to be installed. Right now it's down to the plywood subfloor, and Patty has been looking for errant nails and staples and either pounding them down or pulling them out. It's frustrating and back-straining work, and I bought two extra hammers so our boys can help out. We had a great big pile of trash in the driveway, and fortunately it was hauled away today before it started to rain. I was busy installing networking cables inside the walls of our living room and my home office. My office is empty right now, and all my computer equipment is packed up. I really miss my desk...I'm writing this journal on my laptop this week. It's just not the same.

We took a break this evening and took our kids to the swimming pool at my mom's apartment complex. While we were there, Patty called a flooring contractor that we know and asked him to come give us an estimate on doing our floor. I hope it happens quickly.

Wednesday, June 14, 2017

When Patty got up this morning, she was supposed to take our daughter to cheer conditioning, and our youngest son to reading camp. But the kids stayed up too late last night, and they were whining, and Patty was tired too, so she made the decision to skip the activities and stay home. She'll probably be mad at me for writing that.

She has been preparing food for the coming weekend, when we will be going river rafting and camping in north central Ohio. She's trying to plan out what we will need to eat while we're gone. But with our family, the best laid plans usually go awry, anyway.

Patty and her sister went to two Home Depot stores to pick up the material for our new floor this evening. It's all stacked in the garage right now, and the installer says he'll come tomorrow morning at 8 a.m. and get started. I hope that's not just contractor-speak for, "I'll show up sometime when I can fit you in, and then I'll leave the job half-finished for a few weeks." I desperately want my home office back.

Our daughter took a Sharpie marker and wrote slogans on the plywood sub-floor all over the kitchen today. She is calling it our family time-capsule. Some of it was pretty cute. I took photos, because that's the kind of thing that makes up the family folklore.

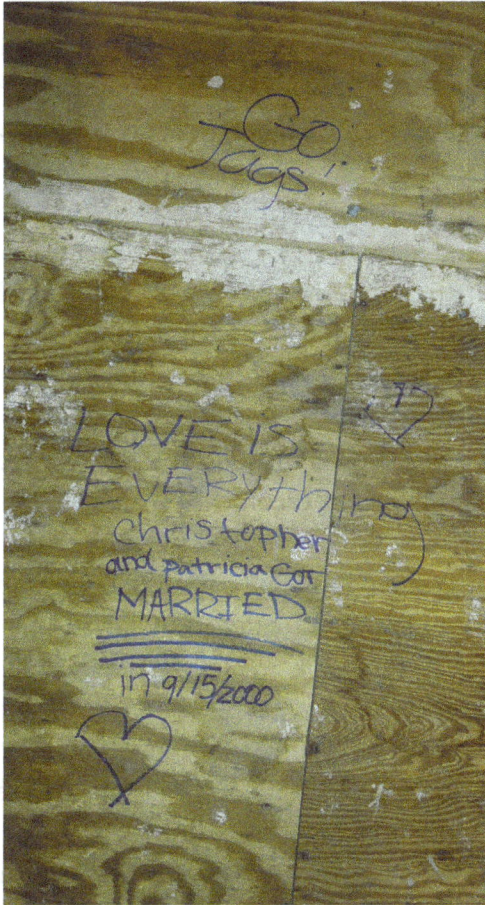

13-year-old Kaitlyn was drawing on the subfloor before the new laminate was laid.

Thursday, June 15, 2017

I woke up this morning to the sound of hammers and saws. I have to say, I'm impressed with the flooring guys my wife picked to do this project. They were here exactly on time, and they got straight to work right away. I left for work soon after they got here and when I came home tonight, the floor was all done. I think it looks great, and more importantly, Patty thinks it looks great too. Having a happy wife gives a man a delightful sense of peace.

That being said, Patty had a rough day. She had to take our kids to their activities, and a neighbor mom had a moving truck blocking *her* driveway, so Patty took the neighbor kid to practice, as well.

Then she was at the appliance store to order the new kitchen appliances that she wanted. She got them all picked out, but then when she went to pay for them her credit card was declined. It was the same credit card she used for the flooring material yesterday. Apparently, the bank has a spending limit within 24 hours and it took Patty almost an hour on the phone with the bank to get it straightened out. That put her behind schedule for everything else she had to do, like picking up the boys from practice, and buying pizza for the flooring guys. She picked up the boys 45 minutes late, and when she got home with the pizzas, two of the flooring guys had already left to prepare for another job.

But at the end of the day, the floor looks really nice. We still have to put on the baseboards and some more window blinds, but it's coming along. What's a little odd, is that our first floor toilet is sitting out on our front porch right now. It's quite a sight.

Friday June 16, 2017

Patty called me this morning, very frustrated that she's still at 237 for the third week now, and she is on a plateau and it really bugs her. She is packing up our bags for our camping trip this weekend and she spent much of the day gathering the supplies we have, and running out to buy the supplies we didn't.

She must have been too busy to log today. She only logged a peanut butter sandwich for breakfast, for 190 calories.

After driving over two hours through some dense traffic, we arrived at the campground about 6:45 p.m. Before dark, we walked along the Mohican River and watched the boys skip rocks. After dark, we built a campfire and roasted marshmallows and made smores, and counted the stars. Patty told me, "I used to be scared to go camping, because I thought I was too heavy for portable chairs...I don't worry about that now. A lot of things change when you lose weight!"

It was good to hear her say that. And she's right. When we were heavy, one reason we didn't like to spend the night away from home is that it was difficult to find a comfortable bed for the two of us. But the bed at the cabin we rented at the campground, even though it was smaller than our bed at home, was perfectly comfortable for us, and we slept very well. It put us in a good mood for the next morning.

Saturday, June 17, 2017

We woke up in the campground cabin this morning, and Patty made some French toast for all of us. She also made sliced bacon in the cabin microwave. Then it was off to the river.

We brought some inflatable rafts to tie together, and we set off in two vehicles to go several miles upstream, and launched our rafts into the river. On the way, we had a momentary scare that we might have left one of our boys behind at the campground, but it turned out he was in the other vehicle, instead of the one we thought he was in. We just couldn't see him with all the inflated rafts.

The Mohican River was fuller and faster than normal, and it was an enjoyable ride. We learned that when you tie a lot of rafts together, they're harder to control, so it was difficult to steer around rocks and fallen trees, and sometimes we just ran into and over them instead of avoiding them. That resulted in a couple of rafts developing air leaks, but they held together enough to get back to our campground.

There was one guy near us that fell out of his raft and into the river. He stood up and started cursing up a storm, because he lost his sunglasses into the river. I was annoyed that he was shouting profanity within earshot of my kids, but I was amused that he was so pissed off about, "LOSING MY OAKLEYS! MY TWO HUNDRED DOLLAR [expletive] OAKLEYS!"

I was really proud of Patty. She had a fun time, and didn't worry about her weight at all. She had a sense of adventure today that I rarely see from her. We were on the river for three hours when we finally reached our campground, and spent another fifteen minutes getting ourselves out of the rafts and the rafts out of the water.

After dinner, 11-year-old Kyle and I played a mean game of one-on-one basketball. He is quite a bit better than he used to be, but since I've lost weight, so am I. It was a competitive game.

Afterward, we all walked from the cabin to Tiffany's camper to start a campfire and make more smores for the kids. The campground had a DJ with a big sound system on this Saturday night, and there was a nearby volleyball court with a bunch of girls dancing and playing volleyball in daisy dukes and cowboy boots. It was a very fun atmosphere, with darkness falling, rows and rows of campers and campfires, country music and fireflies, and the kids roasting marshmallows, hotdogs and smores. Patty was happy, I was relaxed, and it was the kind of summer night that memories are made of.

Sunday, June 18, 2017

Patty got up to make breakfast before it was time to pack up and go back home. She made biscuits and gravy and fried eggs for all of us. She had a couple of eggs and some gravy, but no biscuits. She had a side of watermelon instead. She wrapped a towel around her hand to pull the biscuits out of the oven, because she said there were no potholders in the cabin.

Then, I pointed to the two potholders that were hanging from magnetic hooks on the refrigerator.

After breakfast, we packed up the van and headed home. It was during that return trip that she really said it. She was browsing through Facebook on her phone, and one of her friends had taken pictures of our rafting ride down the river and had posted them on her page. When Patty saw herself in the pictures, she was struck. She was actually pleased. She said, "I don't look half bad in these pictures!" She was smiling. And I was excited about the future. She also said that she regrets shying away from cameras in the past, because she knows she has robbed some memories from our children, and she doesn't want to miss any more of them. It's like she has climbed out of her shell, and then threw the damned shell into the fast, muddy river to disappear forever.

After getting home, we joined a big family Father's Day gathering at Texas Roadhouse with Patty's parents and her sisters, and her aunt Nancy, who had just moved back to Columbus from New Mexico. It was good to see her and her family. She had written a book about a decade ago, and I had just read that book last month. We talked a bit about that, and I let her in on this secret journal I'm writing now, because I wanted to pick her brain about how to publish a book. I'm sure I'll talk to her more about it as the months go along.

Patty ate some smothered chicken at the restaurant, but couldn't finish it and had to take it home to eat later. She managed to finish most of it before bed, and she logged 628 calories for the day. That includes a handful of peanuts from Texas Roadhouse. It really was a great weekend, but it's back to work tomorrow.

Monday, June 19, 2017

Patty weighed herself today, and she lost two, down to 235. I didn't weigh myself this weekend, because we were camping, but I stepped on the scale today. I gained one pound and I now weigh 188. Sigh. Patty is happy with her weight loss again, and she's even bragging to me about it. However, she's very upset that her ankles are still thick. She says she has lipidemia, and her ankles will be thick no matter how much weight she loses.

I think she's nuts. Her ankles look just fine.

Patty and I spent the afternoon tearing down door trim, and then we ran to Home Depot to buy interior doors and register vents. Even though the floor has been laid and looks beautiful, the baseboards are still off, so we can't put our furniture back into place. I miss my home office so badly, I could die. I feel I can't get the most basic things done. I just want to leave the mail in the mailbox, because I really have no place to put it. I heard Patty in the living room shout, "I can't live like this!"

Patty was able to get around in the kitchen enough to make us some chicken wraps. They were very high in protein, and delicious, too. I should have been more grateful for the dinner instead of snapping at her because I was so frustrated with the remodeling disruption. She's just as frustrated as I am.

Tuesday, June 20, 2017

Patty managed to get herself out of our disrupted home to get in an hour of Zumba at the YMCA today. She burned 381 calories, but, as is her habit, she did not eat the calories she earned. She logged only 640 calories today.

We actually made a little headway in the house today. We got the toilet off of our front porch and back into the bathroom, but when I bolted it down, it was still wobbly. I'm thinking the flooring guys just removed the toilet without removing the wax ring, and then I set it down on a new wax ring, and so it can't be bolted all the way down. I ordered yet *another* wax ring, and when it arrives this weekend, I will remove the toilet, scrape off the old wax rings, apply the new wax ring and reinstall. What a weekend treat.

On a good note, we got my home office set up again, and nothing has made me feel better for a long time. I can now get back to journaling on a real computer.

Wednesday, June 21, 2017

Patty took our daughter to cheer camp at a local college this morning. It's an overnight camp, and our girl is going to eat, sleep, and breathe cheerleading for the next three days.

Patty ate a little light today, only 650 calories. She's been saying she needs to eat more each day to get out of her current weight plateau, but if today is a guide, she's not taking her own advice.

When I got home tonight, both of our boys were sleeping in our bedroom. I'm thinking they miss their sister.

Thursday, June 22, 2017

Kaitlyn made a new friend at cheer camp. She sent Patty a photo of herself with her arm around a hunky college boy. She said he is an Ohio State cheerleader, there to help coach the cheer camp. She also called him her future husband. I said the young man is going to have to ask me about that first.

For months now, our refrigerator made awful noises while dispensing water, and the icemaker wouldn't work at all. That all changed today. We had a set of new kitchen appliances delivered and installed, and the old ones were placed in the garage for Patty to sell. She advertised the old appliances on Craigslist, and I'm hoping they will sell quickly, because I can't even get myself through the garage anymore, let alone a car.

Friday, June 23, 2017

I was able to take Kyle to football practice, but when we got there, we found it was cancelled due to all the rain in the forecast. Patty wasn't home because she and Nicholas went to the cheer camp to pick up Kaitlyn. I had to go to work, so I took our son to my mother's apartment, and she took him to get Mcdonald's.

The appliances we had installed yesterday did not match as well as Patty wanted, so we had to go back to the store to arrange an exchange. After that was done, we went up to a nursing home in Marion to visit my friend Charlene and her mother, who was suffering from terminal cancer. Although it was a sad visit, I was very happy to be able to see them both again while her mom was still alive. There were smiles, laughter, and some tears, and Patty showed me once again her natural conversation skills, which I remain jealous of. I'm still amazed at how people seem so comfortable talking to her about sensitive subjects. Hers is a real gift.

Saturday, June 24, 2017

Patty is very frustrated with me today. She has hit a weight plateau, weighing in at 237.4, which means she has been at the same weight for a month. I, on the other hand, have broken my own plateau and lost 3.6 pounds this week. I weighed in at 184.4, which I am logging as 185. She keeps talking about what she can change to lose weight again, and I kept hammering the same advice: don't change anything. Plateaus happen. You're doing nothing wrong. Just stay the course and keep at it. Your body will respond when it is ready.

She was going through her closet yesterday finding something to wear to go visit Charlene's mother in the nursing home. She tried on different things, and she told me today that she might have been too late in doing this. "I have cute clothes that are now too big for me," she lamented.

Yesterday at the nursing home, Patty made a comment that struck me funny. She recounted that one of our friends has a "healthy living" weight loss group on Facebook, and she keeps telling Patty and me to share our weight loss story on that page. Patty dismissed this idea, saying, "nobody cares about *our* story...it's boring." And unbeknownst to her, I'm here writing about it in detail, day by day, in secret.

Sunday, June 25, 2017

We all slept in until after 11 a.m. Patty made us a breakfast of eggs and sausage gravy over toasted protein bread. She couldn't finish all of hers, so I ate the rest from her plate. I used to do that all the time, but since I started logging my food, I usually don't eat from Patty's or my kids' plates anymore. I was sure to log the extra bites today.

Kaitlyn did not eat what Patty made for the rest of us. Instead, she chose to eat cereal and pickles. Cereal…and…pickles. I looked at her and mused, "Hmmm, is there something you need to tell us?" She didn't get the joke for a couple of minutes.

This afternoon, Patty was doing laundry while I was with her in the basement, working on our WiFi router. She looked at me and said, "I want to be skinny like you."

Later this afternoon, Patty and I went to a birthday party for an eight-year-old boy that is a friend of Nicholas. They had the usual summer cookout food, like hamburgers, hot dogs, chips, and potato salad. I had two hamburger patties with onions, and used leaf lettuce as the bun. My niece Jessica thought that was pretty funny. Patty ate half of one of my burger patties.

The party was outside at a community park, and it was so windy that we couldn't light the candles for the cake. The dad cutting the cake had to hold the plates in one hand and cut the cake with the other, so I held the cake container down for him so it wouldn't slide around as he was cutting. That cake looked so delicious, but I knew I couldn't eat any, even though it was literally within my reach. Patty also declined an offer of cake and ice cream.

When we left, we stopped at Subway. Patty had a chopped salad with chicken breast, some of which she ate tonight and some of which she saved for tomorrow. I didn't know what to order, so I checked the Eat This Not That website (www.eatthis. com) for some ideas. According to the site, the best Subway sandwich to order in terms of calories, carbs, fat, and protein is the carved turkey on nine-grain bread. So, that's what I ate. Even though I ordered a footlong, I still stayed under my calorie budget for the day, so I ate without guilt.

Monday, June 26, 2017

I had an appointment this morning with my diabetes doctor. She was impressed with my numbers. I've lost 71 pounds in the past year. Since that time, I cut my blood sugar in half. My blood A1C went from an alarming 10.5 last year to a healthy 5.1 today. My HDL (the good cholesterol) went from 29 to 46. She asked me how I did that. "You can't 'eat' HDL," she said. "You can only get that kind of improvement through exercise."

I don't really do much exercise. Well, I do a lot of pushups. "That'll do it," she smiled. "How do you feel?" Better. Better than I have in...decades.

Later today, we added a family member. Patty took in a three-year-old golden retriever named Maverick, from a local family with a new baby who didn't have room for a 65-pound dog any longer. The kids are over the moon, and the dog seems to like *me*, too. Maverick spent the day getting acclimated to his new home and playing with our three kids. Patty gave him a bath, and brushed out his long hair. Now we have dog hair all over our newly remodeled kitchen. I'll try to stay positive.

Tuesday, June 27, 2017

Patty weighed herself today, she's still at 237.2 pounds, and she's still very frustrated. She had been debating whether or not to go to her Zumba class today, because her foot is hurting her. She decided to wrap her foot in an Ace bandage and go to class.

I had a lull in my work today, so I was able to walk around the shopping mall for 45 minutes. I burned (almost) enough calories to treat myself to a couple scoops of cherry cordial ice cream, which I did. Then work got busy again.

Wednesday, June 28, 2017

Patty is happy with our new dog. *Really* happy. She told me that she is "tears-in-her-eyes" happy, with Maverick's gentle disposition and the way he is fitting in with our home and our family. Last night, she allowed Maverick to sleep with Kyle in his room. By morning, both Maverick and Kyle had migrated to the floor in *our* bedroom. We didn't even know the dog was in our room, he was so calm. She told me that when Nicholas was leaving for reading camp today, Maverick whined and whimpered. The dog has bonded very quickly with our kids.

Patty had nothing to eat today. Well, I don't really think that is true, but she did not log anything today, so I can't tell what she ate.

My sister Amy, a career veterinarian, paid us a visit today to meet Maverick and to give him a checkup. She said he looks quite healthy. And the previous owner had given us his medical records, as well. We've been very fortunate that this dog had found his way into our lives. Patty has outdone herself once again.

Before I went to work, I had to unhook the water, drain, and electricity from our dishwasher, unhook the water from our refrigerator, and remove the power cord from our stove. We're exchanging the appliances we got last week, because the colors didn't match like they did in the store. One thing I *didn't* do is remove the microwave, and when they arrived to take away the appliances, Patty was told that they were "not allowed" to remove the microwave. I was already at work, so Patty called me six times in a row asking how to take the microwave down off the wall.

I'm pretty disappointed in the appliance store. I paid for delivery and installation, and then we were presented with a list of things the installers "weren't allowed" to do. I don't want my wife to order new appliances and then have to scramble to take the microwave off the wall by herself. I want her to be able to sit on the couch with a cup of tea and watch some competent people install her new kitchen.

Thursday, June 29, 2017

Patty weighed herself this morning. The scale read 236.4, or one pound down. She remains on her plateau, and she's angry about it.

Something else has made her angry. She complained yesterday that there was a leak under our kitchen sink, and that I must not have shut off the water when I unhooked the dishwasher yesterday. I was sure I did. Now, today, she complained that there was not only water under the sink, but chopped-up bits of food as well.

A light went off in my head. "Are you using the garbage disposal?"

"Um...yeah."

"Well, stop! It has a big hole in the side where the dishwasher hose is supposed to go. That's where the mess is coming from!"

One group from the appliance store came to remove the old appliances. Patty called me in frustration, saying they nicked the wall, and scratched the new floor. She fixed the floor with some Old English, but it's not over yet…we still have a group coming to deliver and install the *new* appliances. Why does this make me anxious?

Also today, we got a report from our electric company. It told us we're using 16% less electricity now versus last year. I thought about our air conditioning. We don't use it as much as before. We're comfortable at a higher temperature now. Sometimes we leave it off entirely and just open the windows. Our house has central air, but we also have a floor unit that we have used in the past to make it extra cool in our bedroom for sleeping. But I haven't set it up this summer. It's still stored in the bedroom closet. So, we're lighter this year, and so is our electric bill.

Friday, June 30, 2017

This is the second day this week that Patty logged absolutely nothing into MyFitnessPal. I might have to find a way to encourage her, without letting on that I need that information to write this journal.

Patty's ankle is really hurting her today, but that's not keeping her down. She left the kids at home for a bit today to go look at some new carpet for the basement. That is a project we thought we would do first, but it kept taking a backseat to other stuff. Now, we can finally do it.

The appliance truck broke down yesterday, so the new appliances that were *supposed* to show up today did not. Trucks break down, I can understand that. But now we have to wait through the holiday weekend before we can get appliances? They can't just bring it the next day? Yet another reason to be very disappointed with them.

And since we don't have any appliances, we don't have any food in the house, and we can't even heat anything up because we don't have a microwave. Patty broke down and ordered subs and salads to be delivered for our kids. That's really not ideal. Our house has been incomplete in some form for *months* now. It's a tough way to live.

JULY 2017

· · · · · · · · · · · · · · · · ·

Saturday, July 1, 2017

I stepped on the scale with trepidation this Saturday morning. Even though I have not cheated this week, it was one of those weeks I just didn't feel any lighter.

The scale, of course, does not care how you feel. The scale is objective. It can deliver disgust or delight without prejudice.

So, the scale rendered its verdict. I lost two pounds this week. I'm at 182.4, which I'm logging as 183. It's a holiday weekend, and it will be a good one.

Later this afternoon, I saw the guy again. There is this guy, a middle-aged black man, who often walks along Sawmill Parkway and Home Road in Powell for exercise. He's a friendly type, always waving at the passing traffic. I've seen him on occasion for the past couple years now, and with each passing month, the guy has been getting smaller and smaller. I don't know his name, but I'm proud of him. He is inspiring me. And I've started waving back.

Sunday, July 2, 2017

Patty is despairing a little today. She has an appointment with her surgeon this week, and she is still six pounds away from where she was told she should be. I don't think that is a cause for concern, but she is anxious about her doctor being disappointed in her.

Our kitchen still has no appliances, so making food was a challenge today. I had some cereal (without milk) and a McDonald's grilled chicken salad (without dressing.) Patty used the air fryer to heat up some fish and chicken for our dinner. She can be creative sometimes. I don't know what Patty ate today, because she did not log anything.

The carpet installers came out today and installed the carpet in the basement. They did a fantastic job, and they even did it on a Sunday. Within a few hours, our son had taken a bowl of cereal down there. I went down and caught him. He lost his Xbox for a week.

Monday, July 3, 2017

Patty's ankle is still really hurting her. But she still tried a new gym today. Her friend Tina invited her to Planet Fitness to try some sort of exercise that I forgot now. She said she enjoyed it, and she liked the machines they have. I'll have to ask her more about it.

I *did* ask her more about it. She told me she wants to join Planet Fitness, but I'm reluctant. She's already a member of the YMCA, so why does she need to join another gym? We've signed up for gym memberships in the past, and we were always in the 80% or so of gym members who wind up not going to the gym. I'm doing fine working out at home on the treadmill, or walking the neighborhood when it's nice out. That's free.

We got some more frustrating news about our appliances. They were supposed to deliver and install the appliances last week, but their truck broke down. So they were scheduled to come today. By noon, Patty was getting impatient and called them. They said they cancelled the delivery today because, get this—we didn't respond to the voicemail they left us—*last week!* (Who on God's green earth does voicemail anymore?) So now, they have rescheduled the delivery for this Thursday. I insisted that Patty cancel the damned order, but she refused, saying she really wants the appliances.

Life is really getting complicated without appliances, so we spent a little of the time we don't have putting together a hobo kitchen. I set up a card table and put an old microwave on it, atop a pair of scrap 2-by-4's. And we're using an old dorm refrigerator for our milk, eggs, meat, and yogurt. I'm going to plug the hole on the side of our garbage disposal so we can use it again. We're both incredibly frustrated, and we've been sniping at one another. The remodeling is pretty much done (except for the appliances) but we're running into dozens of little details that need fixed, and we never have the right tools or the right parts, or the right attitude, for that matter. Yesterday, I gave up and took a nap, which made Patty mad. Today, Patty gave up and is taking a nap herself, which doesn't bother me at all. That means I get to rant and rave in this journal. I got some more chocolate frozen yogurt yesterday, and I've been eating too much of it again. I've avoided it for weeks, and got my weight down to within rounding error of my goal. This coming weekend, I'm probably going to pay for the frustrated eating.

Tuesday, July 4, 2017

This is not going to be a healthy day for eating, either. The morning was okay. Patty and I both had high-protein cereal. I ate it dry, and Patty had hers with some yogurt. We ate it on the way to the local Fourth of July parade, in which two of our kids participated. It was a hot day, but not too uncomfortable because of our lower weight. We want to do some more fun stuff this summer, like county fairs and carnivals. If our house would ever give us a break, maybe we could.

After the parade, we went across the street to my in-laws' house for a holiday cookout. I overrate, having three pieces of carrot cake in addition to hamburger and chips. What's worse, our neighbors are having *another* cookout this evening before the local fireworks. Like I said, this is not going to be a healthy day for eating, at least not for me. I'd think, being so close to my goal weight, I would double down on my weight loss. But I'd be wrong.

This afternoon, I took Maverick out for a walk in the neighborhood for about 45 minutes. That gave me an opportunity to work off the carrot cake I foolishly ate. When we got home, Maverick laid down on the living room floor, all worn out.

At the other cookout, I ate another hamburger, and some chips and some brownies. Patty ate very little for today, although she did a lot of cooking. I never got to see her sit down, which is sad, because I know her ankle hurts her pretty bad. I noticed that she didn't log anything again today.

Wednesday, July 5, 2017

Back to work, back to healthy eating. Last night at the fireworks, Patty told me she would like to start dancing lessons, but I'll wait until her ankle heals up. We still have lots of little details to do in the house. I've got to put new light bulbs in the basement and fix a drywall goof. Patty finished painting the closet door this weekend and is starting to paint the pantry doors.

We still have no appliances, though they are "scheduled" to come tomorrow. Today, Patty had to fire up the backyard grill in order to boil eggs. She's resourceful like that.

Thursday, July 6, 2017

We got a few things done today in the house. The appliance store *finally* delivered the appliances. They were installed without trouble, and Patty is very happy. We also put the shelves back in the pantry, and Patty painted the pantry doors, and once they are dry, we can install them. Before I went to work, I installed the LED light bulbs in the finished part of the basement. It's nice that things are finally starting to come together.

Friday, July 7, 2017

We were hoping the new blinds for the living room would come today, but they didn't. Hopefully we'll get them tomorrow. Our son has been complaining about not having his Xbox, and even Patty told me I could give it back to him early. But I didn't. I said a week, and I meant a week. He can go out and play basketball, or read a book.

Patty logged very little today, only 420 calories. A ham and cheese omelette for breakfast, and a protein bar for lunch. No dinner. She probably ate dinner, but didn't log it. The scale won't lie.

Saturday, July 8, 2017

No, the scale does *not* lie, Patty lost four pounds, down to 233. She is very pleased, but she wants to get below 230, because she's been in that range for long enough, she says. I, however, *gained* four pounds, to 187. I'm pissed. I know I had the three pieces of carrot cake, and four brownies (or was it five?) but that was back on Tuesday. That was four days ago. I've been good since. It's like the scale is telling me I lost *my* Xbox for a week.

Today we helped our nephew Ryan take away our old appliances from the garage, and now we have some more room for more, well, crap, I guess. It will be really nice to park a car in there one day.

Sunday, July 9, 2017

Yesterday, Patty put together some video game stands for the boys to play their Xboxes in the basement. Later, she went grocery shopping with two of our kids. Our middle boy got his Xbox back today, after serving his week without it. I ran some ethernet cable to the game stands so he doesn't have to deal with wi-fi lag.

Another of my accomplishments: I un-buried the treadmill! Since we finished the basement, I was able to move the futon out of the laundry room. Then I moved the armoire that was blocking the treadmill, which was not easy by myself. Then, I lowered the deck on the treadmill and moved it back into position. It had months of dust and cobwebs on it that I had to wipe off, but I started it up and it works like a charm.

Monday, July 10, 2017

I went out to check the mail, but did not find any. I *did* find a wasp nest. I was stung by two wasps, once on each hand. For me, wasp stings are painful at first, and then they itch for days.

Also today, YouTube taught me how to terminate ethernet cables, so I can make them the right length as I rewire the basement for internet. Patty and I were cleaning the basement, and she pulled out some of her old jackets that we had stored away some time ago. They were *much* too big for her. That made her very amused. It made me very proud of her.

Tuesday, July 11, 2017

We have this new appliance called a Veggie Bullet, that we tried out today. Patty made me zucchini noodles and shrimp... very low calorie and very good! Our kids liked them too, In fact, after the zucchini was all gone, we still wanted more. She also weighed herself today. She is down to 233.

After dinner, I hung the bifold doors on the pantry, and hung blinds in the basement window. There are dozens of these little details to do in the house, and they are going to take forever. Both of us are frustrated, and we sometimes snipe at each other. The place does look very nice, though.

Wednesday, July 12, 2017

Patty called me this morning in a very good mood. She had seen her surgeon, and she weighed in at 230, which is 87 pounds down since surgery. She's been issued a new challenge: to get below 200 lb by the end of November, which is a year after her surgery.

I saw something unusual today. A roadside stand selling funnel cakes! I have seen funnel cake stands at the zoo, and at county fairs, but never by itself on the side of a road.

Now, I have a supreme weakness for funnel cakes, and it took every bit of spine I could muster to just drive on by, but I did.

Discipline sucks.

Thursday, July 13, 2017

Patty spent lots of time in the basement today, going through and decluttering. She had three big trash bags of stuff for me to carry upstairs and throw away, and now our trash can is overflowing. She is also pointing out some things she wants to sell, and having me put that in a separate pile in the garage. My fever dream is to empty out the garage enough to park *both* of our vehicles in it. Today, we can't even park *one* in there. That dream is a long time away.

I just checked MyFitnessPal, and found that Patty did not log today. Maybe she was just too busy?

Friday, July 14, 2017

All of us overslept today. I was an hour late for work. Our son didn't go to practice because neither of us woke him up. Patty has a headache, which she is blaming on her thyroid, and she's had it for several days now. Other than that, it was a beautiful, sunny day.

This is the second day in a row that Patty has not logged any food or exercise. I'm going to have to nudge her.

She found a used kitchen table on Craigslist, and she is sending me up to Delaware to pick it up tomorrow. Then she will paint it and put it in our new kitchen. Years ago, she sent me down to Cincinnati (a two-hour drive) to pick up a bedroom outfit that she found on Craigslist, but when I got there, the apartment reeked of cigarette smoke and the bedroom furniture was banged up and scratched. I knew she would not like it, so I came home empty-handed. I hope it's not like that tomorrow.

Saturday, July 15, 2017

Another weigh-in day for me. I had a good week, and I lost 3.4 pounds, down to 183.6, which I will log as 184.

Patty promised me my Saturday treat of high protein French toast, but first I had to run up to Delaware to pick up the table she bought. My mouth was watering the whole trip back. Then, about five minutes from home, she called me and told me that she didn't have time to cook, and told me to pick up breakfast at McDonalds. I was crestfallen. I didn't get anything for myself there, because nothing could compare to her homemade French toast.

The reason she did not have time to cook was because we had to get dressed for her sister's wedding-vow renewal ceremony. I knew I should not go to the ceremony hungry, because they would probably have food there, and I was worried that there weren't many healthy choices. So before we left, I ate some sliced turkey wrapped around string cheese, and a cup of cherry yogurt. I wanted to get plenty of protein in me so I would not be hungry later.

Patty looks really nice, but she complained that all of her clothes were way too big. She informed me that before our nephew's wedding in September, she is definitely going to buy herself a new dress.

Sunday, July 16, 2017

I finally got my French toast today, but I found out some disturbing news about it. Patty makes this special zero-calorie powdered sugar, using Splenda and cornstarch in a blender. This morning, she had *me* make the powdered sugar. While putting it in the blender, I glanced at the can of cornstarch. Then I glanced at the label. And...I just learned the cornstarch has 35 calories to a tablespoon. I've never logged any of that. I brought this up to Patty and complained...loudly. Patty handed me the plate, and told me, "Oh, it's not going to hurt you. Don't be a baby."

The French toast was good, anyway.

Patty is torturing me today. We're at Kroger, where they are running a sale on 1.5 quart containers of ice cream for 99¢ and she's going through all the flavors, pulling some out, and asking me, do you like this, do you like that? I told her, I'm three and a half pounds from my goal, and *I'M NOT GOING TO EAT ANY ICE CREAM* until I reach it. I know what she's doing. She is still fifty pounds heavier than me, and she's envious. She knows I can't resist ice cream if it's in the house, and she is getting *twelve* containers of it. This is willful sabotage, and I will not tolerate it! (Listen to me, getting all badass and stuff...)

I took Kyle to basketball camp at Otterbein University in Westerville today. I was a student here in the mid-1980's, back when it was called Otterbein College. I showed him the dormitory where I lived as a student. I was hoping that he would stay in the same dorm, but instead he'll be staying in a much newer, nicer dorm that is only a year older than he is.

After dropping him off, I walked around the campus, enjoying waves of nostalgia. I strolled around my dorm, and the Campus Center. I remembered all the fun I had here: the football and basketball games, the blood drives against our rival, Capital University, the morning show I did for WOBN, the college radio station, the late-night softcore porn films on the dorm-lobby TV during the poorly regulated early days of Cable, and sharing scary movies and all-night phone calls with my girlfriend, Mary Jo.

Coincidentally, Mary Jo's roommate, Marty Perry, was the valedictorian of my high school class. When I learned that she would also be attending Otterbein, I thought, "Otterbein must be one hell of a good school if it can land a top scholar like Marty." For my part, I was *not* a top scholar. I was so-so, but certainly not elite. I had a GPA of 3.4 when I left high school. I thought, "So...how on earth did *I* get admitted here?"

During my sophomore year, I was invited to pledge into a fraternity--Pi Kappa Phi, nicknamed, "Country Club." I was one of the very few non-athletes invited to join, and I soon learned that I was in pretty poor condition for the pledge process. The initiations were designed for athletes, with long pre-dawn runs in the snow, pushup contests, wrestling matches in the frat house, and other feats of strength and endurance that left me feeling half-dead. I was sure I would have to drop out, but my fellow pledges kept me going, and wouldn't let me fail. My frat brother and roommate, Mark Reynolds, was my most influential advocate. Mark encouraged me, pushed me, and literally *pulled* me through the final obstacle course in the deep snow, when I was too exhausted to breathe.

Today, I drove by that fraternity house, standing proudly along Westerville's famed "Temperance Row" (a delicious irony in itself), and reflected on those days. I was mostly a bashful and introverted kid when I was in high school, but that experience of being inducted into a college fraternity filled with gregarious, confident, popular boys—and being accepted as one of their peers—gave me a belief in myself that stuck with me into the following years, and especially now.

I started for home, punching up Deep Purple's *Knocking At Your Back Door* (our unofficial frat song from 1985), with a new resolve to succeed at this project I'm on with Patty, reinforced by that little voice, faint but urgent, echoing across the decades from Marty's valedictory speech:

Don't Quit.

Monday, July 17, 2017

And that resolve would be stronger if Patty would just keep all that ice cream out of the house! I'm such a weakling. As punishment, I did the treadmill last night *and* tonight, and I watched two episodes of *House of Cards* while I did it. I'm sure I overate anyway. Thankfully that sale is off now.

As far as I know, she didn't eat any of the ice cream herself. She is just tempting *me* with it. And I'm falling for it.

Tuesday, July 18, 2017

Kyle has been at basketball camp for the last couple of days, and Patty thought she would be looking forward to keeping the house clean for that time. However, Nicholas, the nine-year-old, is picking up where his older brother left off, and he's making a big mess of the place all by himself.

I ate too much ice cream again, but I worked it off by walking the dog, and doing the treadmill while watching an episode of *House of Cards*. Patty sat on the couch, and watched an episode of *The Fosters*, then I helped her tip the furniture over and install anti-slip pads on them so they don't slide around the new floor.

Wednesday, July 19, 2017

I brought Kyle home from Otterbein's basketball camp. He was happy to bring home the camp basketball and Otterbein T-shirt they gave him. He hurt his ankle on the first day, so he had to sit out much of it.

And I ate more ice cream before bed. That was stupid. I'm not going to do the whole self-loathing thing, because this happens to every dieter. But it was still stupid.

Thursday, July 20, 2017

Patty weighed herself at 229, and is very happy she broke the 230-pound barrier.

She ate 715 calories for today. Breakfast was 2 eggs, a slice of cheese, and a tablespoon of peanut butter. She logged nothing for lunch. Her dinner was 4 ounces of hamburger, a little cottage cheese, a little bit of green beans, a quarter cup of pasta sauce, and half of a hot dog. She also had a serving of Cinnamon Crunch cereal for a snack.

Friday, July 21, 2017

Patty did not log anything today, but it was an interesting day, nonetheless. This morning, I took our garbage can out to the curb before heading to work, as it was just starting to rain. By the time I started my van, the rain became a real summer storm, with pounding rain and high wind. I watched the neighbor's trash can get blown over and their trash getting blown down the street. I opened my garage door, and jumped out of the van in the rain and wind to put *our* trash can into the garage so it wouldn't get blown over as well. I got pretty wet in the process. When I got back in the van, I called Patty and told her to take the trash can back out to the curb after the storm blows over.

She didn't remember, and so we missed the trash truck. And since our trash has been overflowing with remodeling trash, that's a real problem.

We also had a real-life crime drama in our neighborhood today. A middle-aged fugitive from Virginia ditched his car in our neighborhood park (where Patty and our neighbor sometimes walk our dogs) and walked across the little bridge to the neighborhood right behind ours. He broke into a house, brandished a gun, and demanded a change of clothes. Then he fled and broke into another house, and apparently fell asleep. The area was swarming with police, with dogs and helicopters, looking for this man. The police warned everyone in the neighborhood to stay inside and lock their doors. Fortunately, the man was caught while napping without anyone getting hurt.

You know what is even worse? I ate too much ice cream again. I wish my kids would eat this stuff so it's out of the house.

Saturday, July 22, 2017

Another weigh-in Saturday for me. Remember all that ice cream I've been eating? It caught up with me. I've gained three pounds, up to 187. That'll teach me.

This was another day Patty did not log anything. She even admitted it. I urged her to keep at it, because "One day, someone will ask you how you lost all that weight, and you'll have a food diary to show them. And you can show it to your dietitian as well. It will be a valuable resource that will help people."

Since we missed the trash truck yesterday, I decided to pull all the trash bags out of our big garbage can, throw them into the back of my van, and drive down to our city dump. It cost me five dollars, and about an hour of my Saturday morning to dump 180 pounds of garbage.

Patty hired a crew to put up our above-ground pool. I was hoping it was too late in the season to put it up, but she was determined. A pool is always more work that one thinks it is, and I was against it. But, once again, I lost the argument.

Patty also painted our railing for the basement stairs. It should be dry by tomorrow, and then I can install it. She asked if it was hard to install, and I said yes. "It has to be a certain height above the stairs, and I have to find the studs to screw it into."

She gave me a sexy smile, put her hand on her hip and told me, "Oh, *I* can find studs…"

Oh, honey, yes you can.

Sunday, July 23, 2017

Once again, Patty did not log anything today. She was busy in the kitchen, though. We had company today; Patty's parents and her aunt, uncle, and cousin, who just moved back from New Mexico. Patty's aunt Nancy is the only one who knows about this journal, and she has kept the secret well.

Something happened that made me feel bad for Patty. We were showing our wedding photos to Patty's aunt. Each of us was around 300 pounds then. Nancy looked at the photo, then looked at the two of us standing side-by-side in our kitchen. She exclaimed, "I can't believe how *amazing* you look, Chris!"

I could just feel Patty's face fall. I sputtered, and pointed at Patty, and said, "But…but…*what about her??*"

"Oh, you look good too, Patty."

My poor wife. I just wish people would make a fuss over her. I can't overstate how much her courage to pursue this surgery has inspired me to lose weight and get healthy. It was never my intention to take the inspiration she gave me and then just run her over with it.

Monday, July 24, 2017

Patty is feeling mopey today. She has a very sore back and a migraine. She admitted she has not been logging her food, and she feels like she just doesn't care much about it anymore.

I took Kyle to football practice this morning, and Patty picked him up afterward while I was working. The coaches gave out the football helmets today, and Patty posted a photo of our son looking intimidating. It was cute. And scary.

Tuesday, July 25, 2017

Patty is even sadder this morning. She actually gained two pounds. She says it's because she is not eating enough protein, and she is not showing enough discipline. I think it's afflicting both of us. I've hit my own plateau this month, as well.

Patty did go to Zumba class this morning. I think it picked her up a little.

This afternoon, Patty, Nicholas, and I went to a local farmers market. I've been under the impression that farmers markets are a place where you can get healthy, locally-grown food. Instead, this one we went to seemed to be a veritable celebration of calories. Sure, there were some fruits and vegetables, and Patty bought some cucumbers. But there were also several booths selling homemade sauces and homemade jams. There were lots of high-carb baked goods for sale, as well as different flavors of raw honey.

There was a truck selling snow-cones, and I was lobbied hard by Nicky to get him a snow-cone. I tried a little apple-cinnamon flavored salsa on a tortilla chip. It was tasty and sweet, but I have no idea about the calorie or carbohydrate load. There was even a prayer booth there, which makes sense because the farmers market was held at a church. I think they would bring in more donations if they had an old-fashioned kissing booth, but that's just me.

Wednesday, July 26, 2017

Both Patty and I have to get up early this morning, because our daughter has to be at cheer practice at 8 a.m., and our son has to be at football practice at 8 a.m., and they're not held at the same school building.

Last night I installed the railing along the basement steps and that, of course, took longer than I expected. So at the end of the night I was frustrated and I just wanted to eat. I ate some Special K high protein cereal and a couple cups of yogurt, and I probably overate for the day. Patty overate too, but only by five calories. I'm glad she got back to logging her food today.

Patty called me this afternoon, complaining of feeling very tired and unmotivated. She says she needs to work out more to get some more energy. I don't know why she calls *me* to tell me that, when she knows she's really just telling it to herself.

Thursday, July 27, 2017

Wow, Patty ate a bunch today. She logged a whopping 904 calories. Two eggs and three slices of bacon for breakfast. One protein bar for lunch. Her dinner was ground chicken with mozzarella cheese and parmesan cheese mixed in. Peanut butter and pork rinds for a snack.

I was at work all day, so I don't really know what Patty did with herself. She didn't call me to complain about anything, so that's a positive.

Friday, July 28, 2017

Patty cooked zucchini noodles and lean ground beef with garlic. It's a recipe she found on a site called Incredible Recipes, and it's called "Million Dollar Spaghetti." But instead of using pasta, Patty used her Veggie Bullet machine to make noodles out of zucchini. It turned out really good.

That being said, it's a shame she didn't log anything today. I keep telling her that people will ask her how she lost all that weight, and if she logs faithfully, she'll have something to show them.

I am home from work today and tomorrow because we were supposed to go camping this weekend, but at the last minute our son decided he didn't want to go, and since it is his birthday tomorrow we didn't want to go camping without him.

Our daughter has given Patty a new obsession on Netflix. It's called *13 Reasons Why*, and she is in the living room binge-watching it right now. I watched the first couple episodes myself, but it didn't hold my interest. Besides, I have this journal to write, and having Patty distracted is very helpful with that.

Saturday, July 29, 2017

Today is Kyle's birthday. The 11-year-old will now be referred to as the 12-year-old. We had a small party for him, with a big cookie cake and some food from Taco Bell.

Patty ate a cantina salad from Taco Bell, but she did not like it, and threw most of it away. She also had a small amount of cookie cake, and actually liked it. The rest of us had tacos, cookie cake and ice cream. Patty only logged her breakfast; a slice of French toast and a couple of sausage patties. She didn't log any of the birthday dinner. Discipline, honey, discipline.

I had a piece of cookie cake, and a lot of ice cream. Actually, it was cherry cordial frozen yogurt from United Dairy Farmers. I just love that stuff. It comes in a 1.5 quart container, and I ate nearly the whole thing. Add that to the French toast Patty made me this morning, and the two cups of grapes and the pile of Doritos I ate for a snack, and I overate by more than 800 calories today.

Discipline, Chris, Discipline.

Before I did all that, I weighed myself when I got up, I lost about half a pound this week, so I basically remained at 187. This has been a bad month for me. I was less than three pounds away from my goal when this month started, and since then I've gained four pounds. I've really gotten off track. I measure my blood sugar each morning, and it has been trending about 30 points higher than it was last month. Instead of a blood sugar reading in the 80s, it's been nearly 120 several times this week. So, beginning tomorrow, I'm going to start taking this effort seriously again.

Patty also weighed herself today, and she remains at 229. She is anxious to get to 217, which will be 100 pounds down since her surgery in November. She has been wanting to join Planet Fitness as a member, and I've been resisting, because we've joined gyms before and we never actually used those memberships we paid for. Tonight, I gave in and told her to go ahead and join. I don't plan to go myself, though. Even though my eating discipline has been slacking these past few weeks, my pushup regimen has not. I still do three sets of 20 pushups every other day, and I haven't missed a set. My triceps are developing well. I've also been thinking of installing a chin-up bar in the basement or the garage, so I can work on my biceps, forearms, and back muscles on the days I don't do pushups.

Sunday, July 30, 2017

I woke up to a screaming match. Patty was yelling at the kids because they don't help her clean the house. The kids were yelling back, which is not okay with me. Nothing sets me off like when our kids disrespect their mother. I've been threatening all summer to remove the cellular data from their cell phone plans. Today I did just that.

When Patty is frustrated, like she is today, she often fails to log her food, like she did today. Nothing. Nada.

As far as myself, I ate more ice cream, which I do when *I'm* frustrated. But I also did the treadmill (while watching an episode of *House of Cards*) and walked Maverick for about 35 minutes.

For dinner, Patty made shrimp, hamburgers and zucchini bake with chicken. I know she ate some of it. Too bad she didn't *log* any of it.

Monday, July 31, 2017

Yesterday, I cleaned out the garage, which generated a bunch of trash. So, early this morning I took a load of trash to the city dump. I got up at 4:30 a.m., And was down there shortly after they opened at 5 a.m. I got back home about 6 a.m., and instead of going back to sleep, I decided to give Maverick an early morning walk. I really enjoyed it, and I think Maverick did too. I'm going to have to do that more often.

I took Maverick for another walk around sunset. This time my two sons came with me. Maverick was more excitable with the boys around than when he is just with me. He kept getting all three of us tangled up in his leash. Also, he pooped on this walk, which he doesn't do very often. I had a bag with me, and I showed Kyle how to clean it up. Now, he's much less enthusiastic about walking the dog.

AUGUST 2017

Tuesday, August 1, 2017

This morning, I found Maverick sleeping in our shower. That was different. He was glad I was up, though, so he could go outside to pee.

Patty called me today, asking me what I wanted to eat on our camping trip this weekend. I really have no idea. She is offering to make my French toast, but that means she will have to take the griddle, and I think we take too much crap to go camping as it is. I'm fine with string cheese and lunch meat.

It's still two more weeks until school starts, and Patty decided not to go to Zumba class today because she didn't want to leave all three kids at home and come home to a big mess. So she stayed at home today. She says she'll go grocery shopping later this afternoon to buy groceries for camping.

Since I'm writing this journal in secret, I can't always write it at home when Patty is there. Today, I'm in a suburban library on one of their computers. When I sat down at the desk, I noticed the desktop computer had no mouse. I had to navigate around by using the keyboard.

Until some clever kid noticed what I was doing, and informed me that I was using a computer with a touch screen.

Thanks, kid. Now I feel old. And stupid.

Wednesday, August 2, 2017

I got up an hour early today and took Maverick for yet another early morning walk. I'll probably do more of this, as long as the weather is nice. It's a nice way to wake up.

Kaitlyn got some disappointing news today. She did not make the high school cheerleading team, at least for the fall quarter. Patty has been trying to console her, and to encourage her to work a little harder so she can make the squad for the winter quarter.

Today is day four of Patty not logging her food. I need to goad her into logging, without her getting suspicious as to why I am so interested in what she eats.

Thursday, August 3, 2017

Patty is in a good mood today. She is wearing her size 14 jeans, which she didn't think she would ever be able to do again. When she started this journey, I think she was in a size 26. She told me she weighed in at 227, which is 90 pounds less than on surgery day. She is happy with her progress, which she hasn't always been lately.

And she logged a snack of peanut butter. I actually watched her eat the peanut butter this evening. She just takes a spoon and digs it out of the jar, then puts it away. Then, sometimes, she'll take the jar out again and have another spoonful. Then she gives me a guilty grin.

"Is that how you count how much peanut butter you eat? Because that's *not* a tablespoon."

"I'm...estimating," Patty replied, busted.

I can't judge. It's not like I don't do the same thing sometimes, especially with ice cream. Besides, looking at her, I can't argue with the results.

I'm also encouraged that she is starting to get some of the same reactions that I've been getting for a few months now. Someone she knew saw her today and didn't recognize her. That made her feel pretty good.

Tomorrow, we leave for a camping weekend. It's also a pushup day for me. I'll have to be disciplined enough to do them while away from home. I'll probably order my chin-up bar this weekend, so I'll have it early next week.

Friday, August 4, 2017

Neither Patty nor I weighed ourselves today, since we didn't bring a scale to the campground, and this weekend we didn't really care.

I've been pretty disciplined with the pushups, but not so much with the food today. We stopped to get gasoline and ice on the way to the campground, and I got a couple of candy bars while getting ice. Then, after we arrived and set up our gear, I ate a couple of homemade campfire pizza sandwiches. I didn't even log this stuff, because I didn't know how.

Patty started to munch on chips as well, but stopped herself, to her credit. She ate half of a pizza sandwich, and then turned up her nose and gave me the other half. Then she had to walk over to the campground bathroom because she felt queasy.

Tomorrow, we're supposed to go tubing down the Mohican River. On the way here today, Patty asked me, "What happens if your inner tube breaks, while you're inside, and loses all its air? How do you get back to your campground?"

"Well, then you have to swim, or walk," I replied. She gave me a smirk.

I felt whimsical, and I didn't stop there.

"I suppose if you had a set of blower cables, you can have someone give you a blow-start. I guess maybe, you'll need to call a… towtube? I don't know, do you have a membership to Triple T?"

Then I exclaimed, "Tubular!" I smiled, as Patty buried her face in her hands.

By the way, I hate taking an inner tube down the river. I much prefer a canoe.

Saturday, August 5, 2017

We woke up to the smell of campfire bacon, and to the sound of river birds. Patty stepped outside the camper and began making some breakfast of French toast, bacon, and scrambled eggs. We had eight people to feed. We had three griddles going, and we even managed to blow the fuse on the camper.

In the afternoon, it was time to set out to the river launch. We tied three inner tubes together, put them in the water and got in, gracefully as ever (not). The river was not as fast as it was the last time we were on it, so we were looking at more than a three-hour river trip.

The Mohican River was certainly crowded this early August weekend! We collided with rocks, trees, canoes, kayaks, tubes, floating coolers, and random driftwood. It was not very warm, and Patty was shivering. The sun was peeking in and out of the cloudy sky. And, although it rarely happens to me, I was actually getting seasick.

I wanted to just close my eyes and let the feeling pass, but you have to be alert on that river, lest you run into debris that can get you stuck. Between the rapids, the smell of stale beer and marijuana, the good music coming out of bad boomboxes, and the intermittent sun and clouds, it was too much for me. I leaned over my tube as much as I could (which wasn't much) and threw up my breakfast into the river.

Patty and our Nicholas were shocked. They didn't even know I was nauseous. I asked for a bottle of water so I could rinse out my mouth and rinse the puke off the side of the inner tube. I felt a little better, but only for a while. After another half hour, the nauseous feeling overcame me again, and I threw up four or five times, getting rid of last night's pizza sandwiches. I made a spectacle of myself, not only to the four others in our three-tube raft, but to everyone else on the crowded river as well. Everyone assumed that I just had too much to drink, but Patty knew I had not had a drop of alcohol for weeks. It's very rare that I get motion sickness, but that river had it in for me today.

We finally got back to the campsite, and after a shower and some dry clothes, I took a long nap in the camper. By dinnertime, I felt much better. Patty cooked some excellent steaks over the campfire, and I ate steak and a salad and some red grapes.

As night fell, I felt good enough to help Patty load some stuff into our van for our return trip home tomorrow. As we walked back to the camper, Patty was shivering again. "I'm so c-c-cold! I think I need my fat back!" she joked.

Sunday, August 6, 2017

Our last morning at the campground. Patty got up a little early, and made egg and cheese omelettes and sausage patties on the griddle. I logged my breakfast, but Patty didn't. I felt much better than I did yesterday, and got my morning pushups done quickly. Then, after breakfast, we cleaned up the campground and Patty sent me to the camp store for some ice and to the dumpster with a bag and a box of trash.

When we left, we took Tiffany and Nina upriver so they could have another river ride today. Then we set out for home, about a two-hour drive. The roads between the campground and the freeway were twisting, turning, country roads. I was driving, and handling them just fine, but both Patty and Nicholas were starting to get carsick. Nicky even started to gag, and Patty hurried to empty her water cup so that the boy would have something to throw up in.

Patty exclaimed that I must have given them both a virus from yesterday, since now both of them were getting nauseous. While I was driving, Patty climbed from the front seat to the back to get some Dramamine for our son. Then she climbed back up to the front seat. I told her I was proud that she could do that, because I know she would not have attempted such a maneuver when she was heavier. She grinned in accomplishment.

We talked about plans for when we are empty-nesters. We talked about selling our house and buying an RV to travel around for a couple of years. She said she used to worry about tiny camper bathrooms, but since she lost so much weight, she feels more comfortable using them. This weight loss journey is changing our lives. Both present and future. I'm feeling optimistic.

Monday, August 7, 2017

Patty was mopey today. She still complained about not feeling well. Nicholas seems to have fully recovered from yesterday's queasiness, so that's good. Patty was planning a big day of housework and laundry, but she couldn't bring herself to do it. Instead, she watched a lot of TV, punctuated by taking Kyle to his football practice.

She isn't very happy with me for some reason . As I was getting ready to take Maverick for a walk, she said I only think of myself. Then we had a phone conversation where she said that I like to sleep instead of helping her. A quirk in Patty's character is that she unleashes complaints about me whenever she doesn't feel good about herself. So, instead of getting defensive and fighting back, I try to make her feel better about herself. Sometimes it works, and sometimes it doesn't.

She didn't log a thing today. I hate when she neglects to do that. Then I have very little to write about.

Tuesday, August 8, 2017

Patty logged today, after my pestering, and she logged 906 calories. I overheard her talking to her best friend Jen on the phone, and Patty admitted to "grazing." This means she's not logging or counting calories accurately. She talked with Jen a long time, and she talked about her weight loss, too, which I hope is helping to keep her motivated.

She also did a ton of laundry today, after saying she would do it all week and procrastinating. So I got to carry six baskets of laundry upstairs before bed. I should log that exercise, from the basement to the second floor, because it was substantial.

Wednesday, August 9, 2017

This morning, I gave Patty a kiss before I left for work. She told me she was going to get up and go work out, and I said, "No you won't."

But it turns out she did. She also told me that she weighed in at 226, which surprised her, because she hasn't been very disciplined these past couple weeks. So, she's in a good mood, and that is good to see after this past week of diet doldrums.

She also had a family scare today. Patty phoned her mother, who sounded wheezy and was struggling to breathe. Patty went quickly across the street to her parents' house and found her mother very lethargic. She called the ambulance and her mother was taken to the local hospital, where they found low oxygen and low blood pressure. So Patty stayed with her at the hospital for a few hours today.

With that kind of dynamic day, starting off high and ending low, Patty neglected to log any food or exercise. I guess I won't pester her about it tonight. I'll wait until tomorrow.

Thursday, August 10, 2017

Patty weighed herself again today, and she's down to 225. She smiled and said she wasn't going to weigh herself anymore this week, because she did not want to jinx it.

Last night I delivered to a bar, and the very cute bartender invited me back for a free drink after work. I did not go back, but it really was flattering. I know, I know; bartenders always flirt. That's how they get their tips. But, they don't always offer free drinks. That one was not what I'm used to.

And it felt strange that I thought more about the calories in that free drink than about the cute bartender who offered it to me.

Today, I had a large chocolate milkshake from Burger King. It has been many months since I've had one of those. I used to drink one or two of those almost every day back when I was, you know, fat. I dutifully logged it, though.

Friday, August 11, 2017

Very little to report today. I'm looking forward to weighing in tomorrow, for the first time in two weeks. I've shown a little better discipline these past few days, and I'm hopeful for a good weight reduction. But, sometimes how you feel is not confirmed by the scale, so it's anyone's guess.

Patty has not logged anything today. Her mother is still in intensive care, and Kyle is sick with a sore throat, so Patty has things on her mind other than logging her food and her exercise. I'll lay off her for now.

Saturday, August 12, 2017

I weighed in at 184, so I lost three pounds over two weeks. Patty says that her father saw her across the parking lot, and he told her that he didn't realize it was her, because she looks so skinny. She patted her rump and said "I don't have a butt anymore!" with a big smile on her face.

Despite these pleasant side effects of losing weight, she is complaining about her hair thinning and falling out. I certainly don't notice it. She was wearing her glasses this morning and I called her my sexy librarian. She's rewarding me by making French toast this morning, my favorite.

I took Maverick for a walk again today. MyFitnessPal says that burns 241 calories.

I'm going to start weighing myself everyday now, because I only have four pounds to lose, and I'm tired of bouncing around, which I've been doing for months. I have got to show some more discipline, and finally get down to 180.

Patty came to a startling realization this evening, after grocery shopping. She said that she doesn't understand why highly-processed, unhealthy food is so cheap, when healthy, fresh food is so expensive. She says it ought to be the other way around. I think I made that argument earlier in this book. But I never shared it with her. So, now, she has arrived at the same conclusion.

Sunday, August 13, 2017

So, I said I would start weighing myself every day, and now I regret it. I gained one pound. It's not fair. I did everything perfect yesterday, and I still gained a pound. I just want to whine.

I installed my chinup bar today. I thought I would start out with 10 chinups, just like I started with 10 pushups a few months ago.

I did two chinups. Two. That's all I could do. And they hurt.

Patty logged only 230 calories today, though I'm sure she ate more than that. Her breakfast was a ham and cheese omelette. That's all she logged.

Monday, August 14, 2017

The scale continues to disappoint. I gained two more pounds since yesterday. I have no idea what's going on.

Patty is scrambling between getting Kyle to his football game today, while still going up to see her mom at the hospital. I hope I'm able to get home early enough that I can help her.

Turns out Kyle did not go to his football game; he went to the doctor instead. He hasn't been feeling well. Later, all five of us went to Wendy's. We remarked that this may have been the first time we all went to a restaurant together as a family in more than two years. Restaurants just are not a thing for us anymore. We went to this one because our niece Brittany works there. I had a grilled chicken salad and a vanilla Frosty. Patty just ate little bits of food here and there, like a bariatric, of course.

On the way home, both Patty and I were singing along to the song on the radio, *More Than Words* by Extreme, to the extreme consternation of our three children.

Tuesday, August 15, 2017

I gained *another* half pound today. I think this is my life going forward. Patty has some good insight that I did not think about. I might be gaining weight because I'm gaining muscle. I've been doing 60 pushups every other day, and this week I started doing pullups with my new pullup bar. Today I can only do two at a time, but I am working on being able to do a third pullup.

I walked the dog and did the treadmill as well. I'm really trying to get back down at least into the low 180s.

Patty made us some steak and salad for dinner today, and it was really great. After dinner was not so great. I got chewed out at bedtime after I pulled a T-shirt out of my dresser drawer that looked unfamiliar . I held it up to Patty and asked, "Is this mine?"

She squinted at it and said no. Then she raised her voice and said, "You need to stop getting so damned skinny." Pointing to Kyle, she continued, "Because I can't tell your clothes apart from *his!*"

Hey, why is she yelling at *me*? After all, she's wearing her 13-year-old daughter's clothes now. What a pair, we are.

Wednesday, August 16, 2017

I finally lost a pound. I did the treadmill and walked the dog last night, and I probably lost a pound of water. But, I'll take it.

Patty is proud of herself for cleaning out her dresser and our bedroom closet. But she only did it because she still can't find her size 14 jeans, and she's really obsessing about it. After calling me and complaining about it all week, I finally asked her to stop telling me that she's looking for her jeans, and only tell me when she finds them.

Patty didn't log anything today. Maybe she was too busy looking for those damned jeans?

Thursday, August 17, 2017

Progress! I lost two pounds since yesterday! Not only that, I *almost* could do that ever elusive third pullup. I'm getting closer and closer.

Patty's mother had to go back to the hospital, and Patty is up there now. She feels overtired and overwhelmed, and I can understand. Needless to say, she failed to log again today. MyFitnessPal has a "bug me" feature, so when it gets really late in the day it will remind you to log your food. At least it does that to me. I wonder why it is not working on her.

Friday, August 18, 2017

I stepped on the scale this morning, and I gained about half a pound. I'm still about 184. Yesterday, another person agreed with Patty's "muscle-building" theory, saying I don't have any fat left to lose. I guess it's a compliment, but I don't believe it. I think I have plenty of fat left. Maybe that's psychological, because the mirror doesn't seem to show it. But I've been overweight for so long, the last place the fat will leave is my psyche.

I have a followup doctor's appointment next week, and I'll ask my doctor about how I calculate my body fat percentage, and where it should be.

I was very naughty when it came to food today. I had a vanilla Frosty from Wendy's, and a big bowl of cereal with yogurt instead of milk, and I finished the bacon egg and cheese biscuit from McDonald's that my son did not eat. Now I won't be able to eat anything tonight, because I'm over my calories.

Patty got her hair cut this afternoon. And then she did something very out of character for her... She took a selfie and posted it on Facebook. It's hard to overstate that. Because for years, she was very reluctant to post any photos of herself on Facebook, and she forbade anyone else to do it on her behalf. So it's heartwarming to see her confident enough to put herself out there like that.

Saturday, August 19, 2017

Patty got loads of compliments today at Kyle's football game. She just got her hair cut yesterday, and she looks *so* much thinner. I think she's entering her "coming out" phase where people who haven't seen her for awhile are really starting to notice.

Nicholas and I took Maverick out for a walk today. But, Nicky wanted to stop at every one of his friends' houses on the way, so we really didn't get any exercise. There were too many pauses.

I weighed in this morning at 184 pounds, and Patty weighed in at 223. That's only a 40 pound differential. When she had her surgery about nine months ago, our differential was nearly 100 pounds, so she's losing weight much faster than I am.

I can still only do two pullups at a time; I've really got to try harder. Patty hasn't logged today again. That makes five days now.

Sunday, August 20, 2017

Patty finally logged something today. She's actually been scolding herself for not logging her food. She ate 600 calories today.

Plus, she is feeling really smug this morning. Earlier this week, she found a new cache of clothes she could wear. And she found them in Kaitlyn's closet. That's right, my wife and my daughter are now the same size. And my 13-year old daughter doesn't know what to make of that.

Patty's mother is still in the hospital, and Patty is heading up there to visit her. She's wearing a T-shirt she got out of our daughter's closet and is showing it off to me with a conspiratorial grin on her face. I told her to hold still for a photo, but she still shied away from my camera.

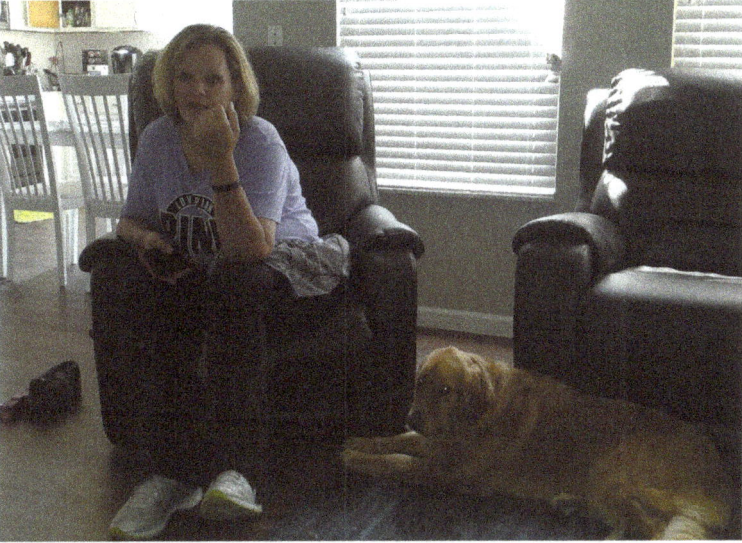

Patty & Maverick at home in the living room. August 2017.

Monday, August 21, 2017

Patty was supposed to go work out at Planet Fitness today, but her workout partner could not make it. So, she didn't go.

We had some new neighbors move into the house on the corner, and they have not one, but *two* golden retrievers. Patty took Maverick over to their back yard to let the dogs run, and they had a good time. Patty got to chat with the new couple, which she loves to do. I was busy hanging the sign above our garage door that lets the world know we have a high-school student in the house. Our freshman daughter is very proud.

Tuesday, August 22, 2017

Patty was very busy today. She took Maverick for a long walk; she measured it at four miles, and the poor dog was exhausted afterward. But Patty seemed just fine with it. She went

189

grocery shopping, too, and found that the FitBit she wears on her wrist does not log her steps in the grocery store, because she is holding her arms on the shopping cart. She feels robbed.

Later, she took Maverick to the pet store to get groomed and his nails trimmed, and he looked much better when they got home.

For dinner, she made some leftover Johnny Marzetti and corn for the kids, and she made herself and me some chicken wraps. She made me three, but I could only eat two of them. I'm not used to eating dinner at dinnertime; I tend to eat it later after sunset.

Since I can't take Maverick for a walk, (he's tuckered out from his long walk earlier with Patty) I plan to do the treadmill and watch *House of Cards*. Patty will watch *The Fosters* tonight.

Wednesday, August 23, 2017

Patty and I had a big fight last night. Probably the biggest one of our marriage. We were putting the kids to bed, a time that I have begun calling "the witching hour," because it gets very frustrating trying to wind down three strong-willed children and a dog and get them all quiet for the night. Patty's cousin from Canada had called, and Patty was trying to chat with her on the phone while we were battling with the kids. Kyle was his characteristic self, goofing off the whole time while disobeying and disrespecting his mother.

Finally, I lost my temper with him. I knew I was going to start screaming at him, but I didn't want Patty's cousin to hear. So I ordered Patty to hang up the phone. She did not. I grabbed the phone from her hand and hung it up without saying goodbye. Then I chased Kyle to his bedroom and erupted at him, yelling at the top of my lungs, losing my voice in the process.

Patty began yelling at *me*, cursing at me for being that rude to her and her cousin, and demanding that I sleep somewhere else. So, I had to sleep on the living room couch, which is not comfortable at all. And all three kids got to sleep with her in our bed. Maverick didn't even come down to keep me company. So, that didn't work out very well for me, did it?

This morning, neither Patty nor I spoke to each other. I left for work without a word. That's really unusual. And it didn't feel good, either.

I *did* stop by the store today and got the protein bread that she likes, and is sometimes tough to find. And I noticed that she has been logging today. She had an egg and cheese omelette for breakfast, and a protein bar for lunch. 450 calories. And she thanked me for getting the bread. We're speaking again.

Today was my pull up day. I can still only do two.

Thursday, August 24, 2017

I had more chocolate frozen yogurt last night, just because it was in the house, and I can't resist it. I stopped buying it, but Patty bought some for the kids, and I just *had* to eat what was left. I didn't even log it, and I should go back and do that right now.

There, I did it. MyFitnessPal says I overate by over 1,300 calories yesterday. Somehow, I don't think it was that much. But the math doesn't lie.

Friday, August 25, 2017

I had to pester Patty to log her food today. I didn't want her to go off on another string of days without logging. She told me when she doesn't log, she doesn't keep track of what she is eating at all, or how much.

Our district manager at work pulled me aside today, and asked, "Seriously, man, how did you do it? What was your catalyst?"

I told him about the MyFitnessPal app. But that's not really a catalyst, it's just a tool. As far as the catalyst, I told him that I decided to listen to my wife. I figured I'll let Patty take the credit this time.

When I got home, I went down to the basement to do some pullups. One of the dangers of putting a pullup bar in the laundry room...I found laundry hanging on it to dry. Sigh.

Saturday, August 26, 2017

I did everything perfect this week...Well, except for the ice cream I had a couple of days ago. But, I gained two pounds. I'm at 186.

Patty and I did some errands today, including some grocery shopping at Sam's Club. We went through the store, with Patty seeing stuff that she thought looked pretty tasty, and then telling me to grab it and read the labels. After a few aisles of this, she complained, "How come everything that looks so good, is so *bad* for you?" We wound up buying some fruit, and yogurt, and bacon, and bottled water, and not much else.

Patty is stuck at about 224, so she's hit a plateau, just like I have. And when she is frustrated like that, she doesn't like to log.

Sunday, August 27, 2017

We have a niece in North Carolina that has announced her wedding for next spring. So, Patty and I have been discussing whether to fly there or to drive there. One thing Patty mentioned, is that we can get more clothes in our luggage, because we're both smaller.

"I could write a book about going from fat to thin," Patty says, while singing to herself in the bedroom. That warms my heart more than I can describe. I'm going to pester her again about taking dancing classes.

As far as the book, I've got that covered. Patty just doesn't know it yet.

Nothing logged again today on Patty's part. I log every day. But apparently, that's just me.

Monday, August 28, 2017

It's my birthday today! I'm 52 years old and in the best shape of my life. Except for being sore all the time, because of the pushups and pullups. But it's a "feel-good" kind of sore.

I had to go to the middle school because Kyle couldn't open the padlock on his locker. Turns out I couldn't either. I had to take a pair of bolt cutters and cut the lock off.

Patty is trying to find some seafood for my birthday dinner, because I love seafood. I told her not to trouble herself. She's looking for lobster or crab, but I told her that I'm happy with shrimp and zucchini noodles. It didn't matter, because she ran out of time to get anything.

Kaitlyn even called me and said, "Happy birthday, stupidhead." Nothing like a little love from your teenage daughter.

We got some ice cream for my birthday instead. I really didn't need that. Patty even put some whipped cream on top. Fortunately, it was fat-free whipped cream.

While eating the ice cream, we watched a TV show called *American Ninja Warrior*. Now, I almost never watch TV, so tonight is the first time I've ever heard of this show, even though it's been on for eight years. I was very impressed with the obstacle courses on this show, and I could just feel the pain the competitors wore on their faces, especially since I've been struggling to do more than two pullups at a time.

Tuesday, August 29, 2017

I did it! I did *three* pullups this morning! Holy smoke, that hurt! Now I have to replicate it tonight.

Patty logged. Let's see, she ate 902 calories. Eggs and sausage for breakfast, yogurt and peanut butter for lunch, ground beef and bacon and cheese and mayo for dinner, and a fudge bar for a snack. A lot of protein today. Good for her.

Wednesday, August 30, 2017

I just listened to Patty on the phone for 20 minutes complaining about everything she needs to do with her days. She has to go to drive-thrus for dinner too often, because she's always on the run and does not have time to cook. She says she wants me to cut back on my work hours and spend more time at home to help her.

While I was gassing up tonight, I overheard a couple of drivers talking about Uber and Lyft. Apparently both of them work for both companies. One driver asked what happens if you get calls for both services. The other driver said he would cancel the Uber run and pick up the Lyft run. I guess Lyft pays better.

Thursday, August 31, 2017

Patty held me up while I was leaving for work this morning, because apparently our son forgot to take his iPad to school today. Each student is assigned an iPad for homework and classwork, and he needs it in class. So I had to run to the school to take it to him.

Patty ate a healthy 900 calories today. French toast for breakfast, some cheese and teriyaki for lunch. (Teriyaki what? It doesn't say.) A taco salad with parm chips for dinner, and peanut butter for a snack. I hope now she is back on the logging roll.

SEPTEMBER 2017

Friday, September 1, 2017

I've been really sore today... In fact, for the past few days. I hope it's not permanent. It's mostly in my shoulders, which have been getting a workout with the pullups I've been doing. I can still only do two of them consistently, although I was able to do a third one last week.

Patty is complaining about being stuck at 224 pounds. I told her plateaus are part of life. But she's really frustrated.

Our seventeenth wedding anniversary is coming up, and I asked Patty if she wanted to go to the Tim McGraw concert at the Schottenstein Center in a couple of weeks. I told her if she wanted to go, she should look for tickets, because I know she is particular about where she sits. She either wants to be on the end of a row, or in the front row of a section, because she has more room that way.

But, she reminded me that she has lost over 90 pounds, and she figures now that she can sit anywhere in the arena and be comfortable. I loved hearing that; I'm really proud of her.

When I got home, she had Luke Bryan music on her computer, and was singing and dancing along. I loved to see her happy.

Saturday, September 2, 2017

Another weigh-in day. 222 for Patty, and she is very happy. I maintained at 186. I'm ready to give up on the goal of 180.

She didn't log very much today; only 267 calories. She made us both my favorite French toast for breakfast. For lunch she had grapes. She counted out a handful of grapes, and asked me, "How do you log eight grapes?" She logged three tablespoons for 19 calories. She's that exact. And then, she failed to log her dinner. I'm shaking my head.

She was so happy this morning, but by this evening she was complaining again about her body. "I'm tired of getting thin because it's really inconvenient. None of my clothes look good. I'm too cold, I get pains in weird places…" So, I guess she's getting sick and tired of winning.

We got hit by Hurricane Harvey today. At least, what was left of it by the time it made its way to Ohio after damaging southeast Texas. All it did up here was give us several hours of a chilly breeze and light rain.

Sunday, September 3, 2017

Patty's Mom was moved out of the hospital and into a rehab center. It's a good thing that she has improved. Patty and Kaitlyn went up to visit her today.

We finally went dancing today! Since tomorrow is Labor Day, she couldn't use the "school-night" excuse. This was a country line-dance class for beginners. I found out I'm even *less* than a beginner. I am really, *really* bad at it. Patty is much better. I also need to go get some different shoes for us, because everyone wore boots and Patty and I had sneakers on. But after months and months of trying, I finally got Patty onto a dance floor. Now, to keep her there.

Monday, September 4, 2017

I had a dream--I was doing pullups and it wasn't a struggle at all. I was doing dozens of them at a time. I was delighted! Then--I dreamed there was a tongue in my ear...

I woke up this morning with Maverick's tongue in my ear. What a weird way to wake up.

We're getting ready for a Labor Day cookout with our extended family. That's going to mean a lot of setup work. And a lot of bad food.

The cookout was more of a success than I had expected. I was right about the setup work. I had to load the barbecue grill into my van, and surround it with chairs and coolers full of food, drinks, and ice. Then we drove two vehicles to the park. It was a nice gathering, and there was no arguing. It was a little windy, and we had paper plates flying around. The kids had fun chasing them down and throwing them away. Then it took about half an hour to clean it all up and haul everything back home. But it didn't rain, and we didn't eat *too* badly. Patty and I shared a piece of cookie cake, and a slice of cheesecake. Otherwise, we ate a bare hamburger and lettuce and vegetables without dip.

Unfortunately, Patty didn't log any of it today.

Tuesday, September 5, 2017

Patty had a rough morning. She had to wrangle all three kids out the door and to the dentist for an 8:15 a.m. appointment. No easy feat, at least with *our* kids. She swore she would never do that again, vowing to schedule them on different days in the future.

Then, when she was bringing them back home, she ran out of gas. She was in the same parking lot as the gas station, but couldn't quite make it. She wound up calling her dad to bring her a gas can, put a gallon in it, put it in her van, so she could drive the few yards to the station and fill it up. She told me yesterday on the way to the cookout that she needed gas in her van. But it slipped both of our minds. It was an interesting experience for the kids, because they have never run out of gas before. I think our boys are big enough to *push* the van, but I wasn't there to make them.

Amid all that excitement, Patty failed to log anything today. Then, when I did my pushups before bed, she called me a showoff. Usually, I do pushups where no one sees me, so I dispute the "showoff" comment.

Wednesday, September 6, 2017

It's Kaitlyn's birthday today, so now the 13 year old is a 14 year old!

When I left for work this morning, Patty was across the street at the neighbors' house, letting our dog run around their yard with their two golden retrievers. Patty was leaning on the fence, chatting with the woman there and another neighbor as well. She used to pretty much hide in our house, not even going down to the corner with the other parents to wait for the school bus. So it's nice to see her put herself out there.

This afternoon we went to Kyle's middle school football game. It was a blowout, 54 to nothing, and we were on the losing end. But Kyle got to start as a defensive tackle, so that was exciting to see. While we were there, Patty ate a protein bar. She stayed away from the hot dogs and pizza at the concession stand, even though she allowed Kaitlyn and Nicholas to eat the junk food. I admire her discipline. I was disciplined too. Bully for me.

At the game, we were both feeling chilly. It's September now, and we're going to need warmer clothes. All of our fall and winter clothes are way too big for us now. Losing weight is getting expensive.

Thursday, September 7, 2017

This morning, I woke up to find Patty in the bathroom, spritzing perfume on herself before taking Nicholas to his speech therapist. I told her she looked beautiful. She held up her hand to me, inviting me to talk to it.

"None of my clothes fit! This hoodie is *huge* on me!"

"Well, let me wriggle into it with you…"

Talk to the hand, again.

"It's not funny! I used to go in my closet and freak out, because none of my clothes fit. Now, I go in my closet and freak out because...*none of my clothes fit!*"

Later, it struck me. Why was she putting on perfume to go see a speech therapist? Maybe I'll have to ask her hand.

Friday, September 8, 2017

Patty's mom left the rehab center and returned to her home today, so Patty spent some time visiting with her and getting her settled in. Later, Patty went grocery shopping and bought more fruit and vegetables. She called me at work to tell me to bring home bread and eggs. On the way into the house, I dropped the grocery bag with the eggs in it, and I could have sworn all the eggs were broken. But when I checked the carton, only two eggs were cracked. The rest were fine. I was glad not to have to return to the store.

I pestered her to log her food today, but she didn't have her phone at the moment, and she did not get around to logging. I have to actively persuade her to keep logging, not only because it helps me write this journal, but because it's a habit we both need to develop in order to keep our weight down. Failing to log your food is the surest ticket to overeating. Modern food, especially highly processed food, has become so tasty and crave-inducing that it's nearly impossible to regulate your consumption just by following the signals your body makes. Food today is designed to defeat your body's self-regulation, so that you'll consume more and more. Logging your food is indispensable. It's as important as keeping track of your spending.

Saturday, September 9, 2017

Another weigh-in day. Patty gained a pound, up to 223. I lost two pounds, down to 185. Despite gaining a pound, Patty is nevertheless in a pretty good mood. She is getting her hair done today; she's having one of her Facebook friends from Indiana coming to do her hair.

Later, she is hosting a surprise birthday party for Kaitlyn at a local trampoline park. A half-dozen of her cheerleading friends are coming to the party. I am going, too, because I had the day off to go to a wedding, but that wedding was ultimately cancelled. So, I have a free day.

Lots of people were visiting us today. Our niece Brittany came to have her hair done also. Another niece, Jaclyn, spent the night with our daughter. We had our nephews Ryan and

Jonathan come by as well, and Ryan brought his stepson Tyson here to play video games with Nicholas. So, we had a full house for most of the afternoon.

Patty took our daughter and nieces to the mall this afternoon. According to the credit card alerts on my phone, they are shopping aggressively. When Patty left, she kissed me goodbye and asked what I thought of her outfit. She was wearing her size 14 jeans, and her Ohio State gear...a size large Block O sweatshirt, and a pair of Block O earrings. (There's a big game tonight against the Oklahoma Sooners.) I told her she was beautiful, and I commented that you can see more of her neck and shoulders than you could when she was heavier. And I told her she looks sexy from the rear, too. She gave me a teasing scowl as she walked out the door.

She called me from the mall, kind of emotional. She's been trying on clothes with the girls, and she was struck by how many more kinds of clothes are available for her. "I've always had to shop in the fat stores, and now I can shop *anywhere*. Everything looks so cute. And I can't buy everything that looks cute! There's too much of it!"

I'm really, really proud of my wife.

Sunday, September 10, 2017

And I'm really, really disappointed that our Buckeyes lost the game last night to Oklahoma, 31-16.

I had a dream last night that there was a wedding at our house, but I didn't know the couple. And it was a chinup day for me, so I was trying to find an opportunity to sneak down to the basement to do them. A bunch of kids were down there making a mess of things. There was laundry hanging on my chinup bar. Then, when I grabbed the bar, it came right down off the steel beam it's attached to. The mount had broken, and I thought I'd have to return it to Amazon. It was a typical type of dream that lots of people have; a cascading list of frustrations where nothing is going right.

The weather in Ohio today is calm, sunny, and warm. However, there is a massive evacuation going on in Florida, because of Hurricane Irma. Millions of people are clogging the roads, trying to get to safety, suffering a cascading list of frustrations that is very, very real.

Monday, September 11, 2017

I saw my family doctor today. He's the one that first diagnosed me with diabetes, and told me of the bad things that will happen to me if I didn't get control of it. Today, he was gushing about me to the young medical intern that was with him. He also told me that whenever he sees my wife, half of that appointment is her complaining that I'm losing more weight than she is and that I'm looking better than she is. He thought that was amusing. Looking at my numbers, he adjusted my prescriptions (for my lower weight), pronounced me perfect, and told me to come back in six months.

Oh. When talking about the exercises I do, he told me *he* couldn't do many pullups either, despite trying. So I'm not alone.

I'm looking forward to some of the milestones that Patty has yet to reach. She started this journey at 317 pounds, and has lost 94 pounds so far. Soon, she'll reach that 100-pound weight loss mark. Later, she will break the 200-pound barrier and enter One-derland. After that, she'll fall below my weight. I think that's the milestone she's looking forward to the most.

While eating dinner tonight, Patty was telling me she needed to make a dessert for Kyle's football team. She wants to make Oreo truffles, and she said she would have to do it while the kids were in school and while she has tape over her mouth.

She said that after her surgery, she would get sick if she ate chocolate. But now, she can not only tolerate it, she can crave it. She recognizes that that can be dangerous, so she is thinking about just buying some cookies at the store for the team instead of filling her kitchen with the truffle temptation.

Tuesday, September 12, 2017

After several weeks of no treadmill, I did an hour on it today. Usually, when I'm home, I'd take the dog out for a walk, but it was raining, so I did the treadmill instead. I watched an episode of *House of Cards*, one that I think I watched before.

Patty did a lot of dollar store shopping and outlet mall shopping with her niece and her mother today. Her mom has been cooped up in the hospital and rehab for weeks, so it was nice for her to go out shopping.

Once again, Patty neglected to log anything for today.

Wednesday, September 13, 2017

Patty did not make Oreo truffles today, but she did make cookies. This morning she sent me to the grocery store to get her some chocolate chips and some M&Ms. On my way to the store she called back and told me to get Mini M&Ms. Then she called back and told me to get regular M&Ms Then she called back a third time to tell me to get Mini M&Ms, and to get two bags of them. I know it's a woman's prerogative to change her mind, and my wife is a woman of prerogative.

Later, she called me to say that she made all those cookies and she avoided eating even one of them. So, she was proud of herself, and I'm proud of her too. She took the cookies to our son's football game, and she was a big hit. Hopefully the players might even treat my son well, because he has such an awesome mom.

While at the store this morning, there was a bag of almond M&Ms, which I have never tried before. So, I got a bag. And I ate some. Then I ate more. Then I ate the whole damned bag. Over 1,300 calories, which I didn't need, but they were good. Forgive me, journal, for I have sinned.

Thursday, September 14, 2017

I've been pestering Patty about logging her food, and today, she told me that she was trying hard to do it. The idea of logging food, of course, is to prevent yourself from overeating, or at least from overeating by accident.

Tomorrow is our anniversary, and I have the night off work, so we're talking today about what we should do. Since having kids, it's been very rare when we have a night out to ourselves. And since we don't really go to restaurants anymore, we have to be more creative in finding something to do with ourselves. We talked about walking around a mall, or going to a comedy club, or going to a bar to see a band. We haven't decided on anything yet.

Friday, September 15, 2017

We were still making several plans for our anniversary today. We were going to go to a high-school football game, which we have never done together. But, then we were talking about other plans. We were going to go to a Japanese steakhouse. But, the people Patty wanted to come along decided not to go. We were going to go to a sports bar with Patty's friend whose boyfriend was a DJ there. But the friend came down with a sinus headache and decided not to go.

We wound up going...nowhere. What a boring anniversary. We both agreed that I should have gone to work. The only thing that was accomplished was that I assembled the combination dog cage/end table that Patty ordered last week that has been sitting in my office in the box for a few days. It was a very complicated thing to put together, too. Maverick seems to like it okay. He won't go into it on his own volition, but he'll go in there if we tell him to.

Saturday, September 16, 2017

That overeating on Wednesday ruined me. I gained 3 pounds, now I'm up to 188. But my jeans aren't any tighter. My T-shirts *are* tighter, but not in the belly. They're tighter in the chest and arms. I'm frustrated about the weight, because in the MyFitnessPal app, when you complete your log for the day, the app will tell you what you will weigh in five weeks if every day were like the day you just logged. For me, each five-week projection is below 180 pounds. (One day, it was 169.) But I never, ever, get there. I've been stuck in the 180s, literally, for months. I dropped below 190 pounds back on April 22. Five months later, I'm at that same weight.

Patty has lost a couple pounds, down to 221. She's happy about that, but she's very disappointed in her loose, flabby skin, especially on her upper arms and around her belly. She was stripping down to take a shower today, and was showing me her problem areas, in total frustration. I was showing her my own problem areas, too, and she smirked at me and said, "Really?"

She says I don't have any problem areas. I told her I never have seen her more slender than now, and that nobody sees the details on her; they only see the big picture, which is a much smaller picture now. That didn't cheer her up, though.

Sunday, September 17, 2017

This morning, a little after 7 a.m., I was awakened by the phone ringing. It was Patty's dad, and he needed help with Patty's mom. Usually he would call Patty when her mom needed help with dressing or bathing or housework. But in this case, she fell off the bed and he needed my help picking her back up. So, I put on some clothes and walked across the street, barefoot. When I got there, we were about to pick her up, but she was complaining about her back hurting and she wanted us to call the paramedics. So, we did.

The Columbus Fire Department was swift and professional, and they got her up off the floor and into her wheelchair. They also checked her blood pressure and blood sugar, and made sure she was uninjured, lucid and safe in the house.

I was thinking a lot when I returned home. Patty's mom had her stroke when she was younger than I am now. She's a good woman who raised four daughters, worked at a bakery, and kept her family fed and clothed and her home cleaned. Even after her stroke, while she could still walk somewhat, she was always the first to help Patty clean the kitchen when she visited us, and she watched our kids, if she could, when they were younger. She doesn't deserve the medical problems she has. If anyone deserves them, I thought, it was me.

I've been fortunate that I've been able to avoid the abuse of alcohol and tobacco during my life, not because of any supreme discipline, but because I just didn't enjoy either. I did, however, abuse my body with unhealthy food and general laziness for decades. In that way, I've been thoughtless and selfish, putting my health and my family's future happiness at risk. There's no reason I shouldn't have been helped into that wheelchair myself this morning. There, but for the grace of God...

At times, I think that I must be dreaming. That I'm really a helpless invalid, and that my loved ones are burdening themselves taking care of me. That I'm in some drug-induced dream world, where I'm young and healthy and strong. What would I do there? How could I enrich my family's lives? How could I make my wife happy? How could I make my mom proud?

When I came back through my door, I got down on the living room floor and did my twenty morning pushups. Then I returned to bed and cuddled with my wife.

When she got up, she made all of us some very tasty omelettes with ham, cheese, mushrooms, onions and peppers. Toast and jam too. Later, we went to our youngest son's flag football game with our neighbor, Kim.

Last night, I was hoping to take Maverick for a walk, but Patty's dad called Patty over to their house to help with her mom. He didn't specify what kind of help she needed. She said she'd be gone for five minutes, but she was there for over an hour. I put the boys to bed, so she wouldn't have that to worry about when she got home. She was going to pack their lunches before bed, but decided against it. Needless to say, I didn't get any exercise tonight.

Monday, September 18, 2017

Patty's mom returned to the hospital today with pneumonia. Patty was hoping to get a lot of housework done today, but instead she had to run up to see her mom. She called me this afternoon with a list of errands for me to run, like picking up medicine for Nicholas and then picking up Kyle from football practice. Then I'm supposed to go to McDonald's and get dinner for the kids. I have some of my own errands to run too, and I don't know if I'll get them done. It's a very busy day for both of us.

Too busy, I guess, for Patty to log anything. I logged *my* stuff, though. I haven't missed a day yet.

Tuesday, September 19, 2017

Patty was sure grumpy today. I left early this morning, so she had to get the kids ready by herself even though she was hoping to have my help. As soon as I got home, she told me to unload the groceries from her van because her back was sore.

Later this evening, she was sore at me because I went to my mom's apartment to help her set up a TV antenna. Apparently, AT&T U-Verse is having (another) contract dispute with our local CBS station, so Mom can't watch the CBS shows that she likes. She can watch them here at my house, so she asked me what cable company I use. I told her I don't. I haven't had cable TV for the last six years. I have an antenna attached to the back of the house, which is connected to our TiVo box so we can record shows. We can also watch Netflix, Amazon, and YouTube through the TiVo. I told Mom she could get a cheap antenna and watch the local CBS station through that, although she couldn't record it. She liked that idea, so I went to the store, got a $20 antenna, and went to her apartment and hooked it up.

Note to TV executives: Grow the hell up. These contract disputes are childish. *I'm* pretty much immune to them, since I stopped watching TV years ago. I read books instead. (And right now, I'm writing one.) But when you inconvenience my beloved mother, you get my temper up. I see each side shouting from the mountaintop about how they are only thinking about the 'customers', and then when they finally agree on a contract, it means the customers get rewarded with...higher cable bills. Work out your dumb contract *before* it expires, and skip the brinksmanship. It makes you all look foolish.

Wednesday, September 20, 2017

Patty told me she is planning our annual football party for the end of this month. Every year, on a Saturday when Ohio State is playing a night game, we make a bunch of food and set up a TV projector to show the game on our garage door for the neighborhood. It's become quite a hit.

I'm going to have to spend some time this weekend getting all the connections together to feed the projector, to get the sound speakers set up, and to decide what food and drinks we need. I hope to make my steak-sauce based chip dip, which the neighbors seem to like. We had one party get cancelled last year because of rain, so I hope it doesn't rain this time.

Three days in a row that Patty didn't log her food into MyFitnessPal. Next time she complains that she isn't losing weight, I'm going to point that out to her.

Thursday, September 21, 2017

Before I left this morning, I helped Patty make the bed. There was a commercial for the US Army playing on the radio.

I told her, "Maybe I could join the Army now...but, no...I'm way too old."

She said, "And I'm way too fat."

"No, you're not!", I said.

Then she said, "I'm jealous of those people who have it all together. I need a life coach..."

"Um, no. You could *be* a life coach. You're the most productive woman I know. And you're mine, all mine!" I hugged her and made naughty promises and went to work with a smile.

This afternoon, Patty called me, all excited. She had just left Kyle's football game. Kyle got to play center, which is a position he'd been wanting to play all season. According to Patty, he did really well. We're both really proud of him today. I was told he's bringing his grades up, too.

Friday, September 22, 2017

Today was better. Patty logged a full day, 725 calories.

I was very busy at work today, and I got very little sleep. Patty called me a few times to check up on how I was feeling, and she told me to go straight to bed when I got home. We have a wedding to attend tomorrow, so she said, "Just skip whatever you do on your computer when you get home and go right to bed!" She doesn't know yet what I'm doing on my computer. I take notes on my phone through the day, and then I write my journal entries when I get home.

Saturday, September 23, 2017

Patty let me sleep in, while she took her niece to get their hair done for our nephew Ryan's wedding today. She went to one place, but the wait was too long so they wound up going to another salon for their hair. On her way home, she called me to wake me up and to get our sons into the shower and to start getting them dressed.

The first thing I did was to weigh myself. Still 188, although I lost about half a pound. I've accepted this new reality, that as long as I'm doing the pushups and pullups, I'm just replacing fat with muscle and I'm not going to lose any more weight. In fact, I'll probably *gain* slowly. I've still got to go and get my body fat percentage calculated. I'm very interested in that right now.

We went to our nephew's wedding today, and it was a lovely one. Patty received plenty of compliments on her looks, which made her happy. This time, people made more of a fuss about *her* than about me. She even got up to dance a few times, and she had some wonderful photos taken of her. I got to talk to our Aunt Nancy, an author herself, about this journal I'm writing and how to get it published. Patty almost caught us. She asked, "What are you two talking about?"

I replied, "Losing weight." It wasn't a lie, really.

There was a very touching moment at the reception. During a slow dance, Patty's dad took her mom to the dance floor in her wheelchair. Her mom removed her oxygen mask, and allowed her nephew, the groom, to pick her up out of the wheelchair. She held on as tight as she could and stood on her one good leg...and she danced with her grandson, to the tears and applause of everyone there. It was the most remarkable moment of that wedding reception.

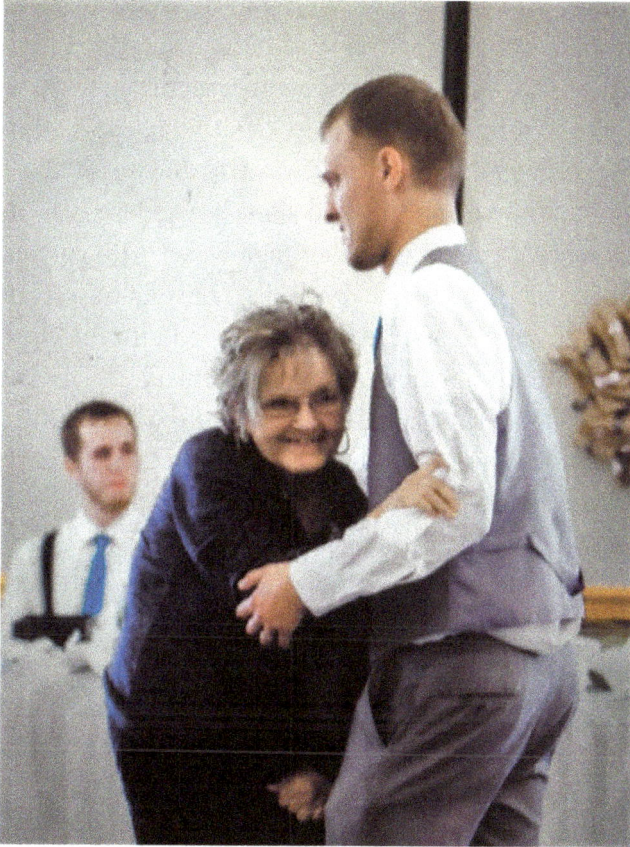

Patty's mom Linda, dancing with our nephew Ryan at Amanda & Ryan's wedding reception.

The food was okay. We had roasted chicken, green beans, and salad. Well, that's what Patty and I had. There was plenty of other food, but it was carb-based stuff like rigatoni and potatoes, which we avoided. I did have a couple small slices of wedding cake, which was good. Patty had just a forkful of cake, and told me it gave her tummy cramps.

As the night wore on, I was getting a little anxious. I had to find a place to do pushups. I did 20 of them when I got up, and I usually do another twenty around dinnertime. But it was after 7 p.m. and I still hadn't done my second set of 20. I don't like to do them in front of people, especially people who don't know I do them already. And I was wearing a suit and tie, so that would really be an unusual sight. I wandered around the reception hall, and spotted a storage closet with just enough room to knock off a set of 20 pushups. I haven't missed any yet, and I didn't want to start now, so I slipped into the closet and got on the floor, knocking them off in a hurry.

Once again, Patty failed to log anything. I've really got to pester her some more. Kaitlyn has her cousin Jaclyn staying at our house for the weekend. They're making "slime" out of glue and laundry detergent. Kids.

Sunday, September 24, 2017

I was awakened to a locked bedroom door and a suggestive grin on my wife's face. "Opportunity knocks!" she teased. There's nothing like a wedding to get a lady into a loving mood…

Afterwards, Patty made us all an awesome breakfast of french toast and eggs and bacon. After I ate, I flopped down on the couch because I was still tired from a long week. I got up later to go to Nicholas' flag football game, and some time after that I went back to my mother's apartment to fix her TV antenna again, because the local CBS station stopped coming in. I had to launch the TV into another channel search to find the station again.

Patty spent a lot of time with her mom across the street. She is back home after being in the hospital, and Patty was over there writing down the medications she needs to get from the pharmacy and to get her settled in. So, Patty didn't make dinner, and I let the kids eat mac and cheese and cereal and pretty much whatever they wanted.

I was planning on walking the dog, but I didn't want to leave the kids alone to mess up the house. I wanted it picked up and presentable when Patty walked in. I emptied the dishwasher and picked up blankets and pillows out of the living room. Then I went through the house and gathered all the trash because the trash truck comes through the neighborhood tomorrow.

Monday, September 25, 2017

Patty has a bad headache today. She is calling it an allergy headache, but she couldn't find her allergy medicine. Instead, she took migraine medicine, hoping that would help. Her back also hurts, and she asked me to rub it this morning. She says it's a common problem for bariatrics to experience back pain, which is counterintuitive to me. I thought the weight loss should make you feel better, not worse. I will say that Patty never goes to the hospital anymore. She used to have to go to the emergency room three or four times a year with debilitating back pain, which only rest and a pain shot would remedy. But that hasn't happened since her surgery, so that's a marked improvement.

We went to Kyle's football game this afternoon. He was playing center last week, his favorite position, but today he played defensive tackle. His team won, 6-0. Then, we went to McDonalds, which I still think we do too often.

This evening we were setting up for our Buckeye party this Saturday night. I've been getting the cords and cables together, and the projector and speakers ready. It was a pretty night to spend on the driveway testing everything out. I'm thinking our speakers aren't loud enough, and we might go tomorrow to get more.

Tuesday, September 26, 2017

I had to listen to a lot of Luke Bryan today. He has a song called *Strip It Down*, and Patty was watching the video for the song on the living room TV over and over and over.

Patty told me tonight that she's going to try to do a better job logging her food. While she was eating, she was logging her dinner, and she kept asking me to get up and grab the can of roast beef and the can of gravy off the counter so she could scan the barcode into MyFitnessPal.

Later, we went grocery shopping at Sam's Club, mostly for junk food that we're going to have at the Buckeye party at our house this weekend. We got chips, hamburger buns, cream cheese, and bottled water. We got some single serve potato chips that Patty uses to pack lunches. We also got some seedless grapes for ourselves.

And, I got a great big 100-watt Bluetooth speaker for our party. I'm looking forward to it.

Wednesday, September 27, 2017

I did not see much of Patty today. It was a shopping day for her, She and her aunt Nancy and her cousin Lisa went down to the Jeffersonville Outlet Mall, about 90 minutes away, to spend all of our money.

They went to have lunch at the Subway in the mall, but when they got there, the Subway was no longer there. In its place was a Chinese restaurant. Patty settled on a little bit of teriyaki chicken. She found out later that the Subway wasn't gone, it had just moved to another part of the mall. She asked why the Chinese restaurant didn't tell her that, and I said, "Why would they? They might lose business that way."

She's not committing to logging; there was no record of today's eats.

Thursday, September 28, 2017

Patty finally got the orthotic for her foot that she's been waiting on for weeks. She's only supposed to wear it for a couple hours the first day, and then gradually wear it more as time goes on. I asked her if she'll be able to go to dance class this Sunday night, now that her foot is fixed. She cocked her head at me and said, "Um...No."

I don't want to give up on her. I don't want to give in. We have 11 nieces and nephews, and the first one just got married last week. Another one will get married this coming April. I expect more will soon follow. There will be lots of receptions coming up, and lots of opportunities for me to dance with my wife. I have a vision, and I want to see it through.

Patty saw her doctor today to get the orthotic, and she had some blood results come in. Her thyroid numbers were extremely high, and that's why she has been so tired lately. She said she needed to take a two-hour nap yesterday after shopping, and she really wanted to do the same today. I guess I'm glad there's a medical reason for her fatigue, but I'm thinking it's more because of all the work she takes on, between the house and the kids and the dog and her mom. A pill is not going to help with that. The Rolling Stones tune, *"Mother's Little Helper"* just popped into my head. Now, if you're old enough, it's in *your* head, too.

She did manage to log her food today. A total of 860 calories for the day. I hope that will give her some more energy.

Friday, September 29 2017

Patty did a lot of food prep today. She made a bunch of no-bake cookies and a bunch of chocolate and peanut butter buckeyes for the party tomorrow. She called me and told me that she was proud she got it all done, and she was even more proud that she didn't eat any of it. Now, she says her mission is to keep the kids out of them until the game tomorrow.

She only logged her breakfast today. 168 calories of peanut butter and a small banana. If that's all she ate while baking cookies, she's got the discipline of a monk.

Saturday, September 30, 2017

We each lost a pound. Patty is at 221, and I am at 187.

It was a great day for our Buckeye party. Patty and I each made some dip; she made buffalo chicken dip and I made my steak-sauce dip. She gave me a quick haircut, and then sent me to Sam's Club for cupcakes and chips and other party food. Others were bringing hot dogs and hamburgers, and our neighbor Tino had taken on grill duty.

This is the fourth year we've done this party, and it gets bigger every year. We were expecting about 50 people from the neighborhood, but we easily doubled that. Patty's sister said there were about 125 people there by kickoff. We did something a little different this year. We hired a woman who does face painting for the kids. This was the same woman who brought the Easter Bunny to our easter egg hunt a few months ago. She was mobbed by dozens of kids in the sunlit hours before the game. Patty even got a Block "O" painted on her left cheek. Neighbors kept showing up with pies and deviled eggs and more chips and snacks. Many of the neighbor boys played a pick-up game of basketball on our hoop out by the street. Other kids were zooming up and down the cul-de-sac on scooters and bikes.

About an hour before the game, Patty sent me to Roosters to pick up an order of 100 chicken wings. I didn't mind doing that, but I was concerned that with so many people showing up, I was going to lose my parking space. My mom drove up, and after seeing all the little kids running around, called me over to her minivan and asked me to park it for her, because all the active children were making her a bit nervous, especially about backing into a parking spot. We didn't plan on our party being such a draw for kids, but that's what wound up happening, especially with the face painting and cupcakes we were offering.

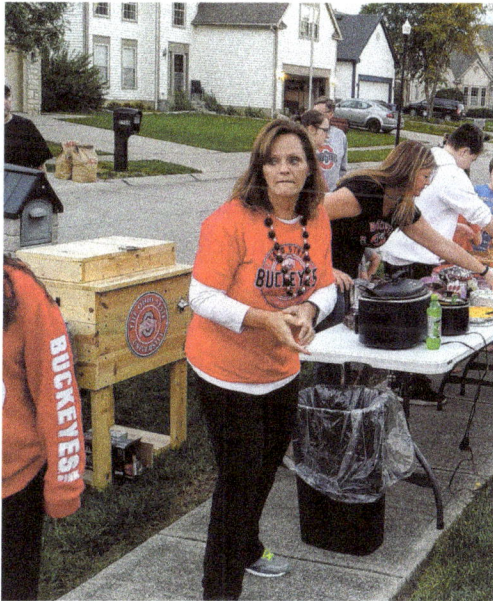

Patty working the neighborhood Buckeye party.

The sun went down and we all set up our chairs on and off the driveway to watch Ohio State take on Rutgers University in New Jersey. We were projecting the game onto our garage door. The game became a blowout early, with the Buckeyes leading 35-0 at halftime. That was actually a problem.

When the sun went down, the autumn chill came into the neighborhood pretty strong, and not everyone was dressed for it. Also, the parents who brought their kids had their hands full with worn-out, chilly kids. Add all that to a not-very-exciting football game, and the party disbanded quickly. Almost everyone had left during halftime, and the ones that were left had stopped watching the game and were helping to clean up the yard and the trash off the tables we had set up.

Despite ending early, the night was eventful. My friend Angie got hit in the head with an errant basketball while she and her husband Eddie were walking to their car. We learned that one of the neighborhood teenagers made off with a can of beer while no one was looking, and Patty wasn't happy about that. The projector flickered out a couple of times, which wasn't too big a deal since the game wasn't close, but still. We were cold and tired, and decided to just move the tables and coolers into the garage and clean it up tomorrow. So, after throwing a party on a Saturday night for over a hundred people, we managed to get into bed somewhat early.

Patty did not log anything today. I knew she was sampling some of the food people brought, because she complained about feeling queasy. (Not that the neighbors bring bad food; they don't. It's just Patty can't tolerate rich, sweet stuff.)

OCTOBER 2017

Sunday, October 1, 2017

I added a pushup to each set today, so I'm doing three sets of 21 pushups every other day. My plan is to add one per set every month until I'm doing three sets of 25, for 75 pushups every other day. On the other days, I do pullups on my basement pullup bar. I can usually do three pullups now.

Instead of spending the day cleaning up from the party, we decided to spend the day at the Columbus Zoo. We took Patty's mom and her wheelchair with us, and a bunch of other extended family. We rode the train, fed the giraffes, and saw some newer exhibits. We got plenty of exercise walking around the zoo, too. Kyle found a penny, and bent to pick it up. Then he jumped back, and said, "That's not a penny...it's a squished Skittle!"

Patty told me how she used to have a hard time getting onto the zoo train. Now, it's very easy for her. Another benefit of losing the weight. She still complains about body aches, but she is growing into her new physique day by day.

We did not eat at the zoo. The food is too expensive and not very healthy. The family decided to go to Golden Corral, which presented Patty and I with an unusual dilemma: how do restaurants fit into our lives now? We wanted to spend time with family, but Patty can only eat a Dixie cup full of food at any one time, and it's a buffet-style restaurant that costs about $15 per person. That would be expensive to feed the *both* of us, given what we eat now. I had some imitation seafood salad on a bed of romaine and some cubed fruit. Patty ate a little salad with some chicken, and we even shared a tiny cup of soft-serve ice cream. Our boys ate like...boys. So, maybe we got our money's worth because of *them*.

Monday, October 2, 2017

Patty got weighed in at her doctor today. She lost two more pounds; she is at 219. She has been complaining about feeling exhausted all day. She says she's missing something, something that would give her energy. I couldn't help it. I said, "Umm… food?"

The doctor wound up adjusting her thyroid medicine to help with her energy level. When they were discussing her weight loss, the topic turned to *me*. Patty told her doctor that I made her journey easier for her. That was truly touching.

Her mom is back in the hospital. It's hard for Patty to make plans with me or with the kids, because she feels "on-call" whenever her mom is in the hospital, or even at home for that matter.

She was at the hospital with her for a few hours this evening, and I told the kids to have the house picked up and their teeth brushed and to be in bed when she walked in the door. I wanted nothing in between my exhausted wife and her warm bed. I had to turn off the Wi-Fi in the house to get the kids to move it, but it finally worked.

Tuesday, October 3, 2017

I finally cleaned up the garage from our football party this weekend, and I took several bags of trash to the city dump. Now, Patty can park her van in the garage once again.

Work ran long for me today, and I had to get an oil change, too, so I was late getting home. When I got there, Patty told me we had to run to the store to get some khaki shorts for Kyle. His football team was going to wear them to school. Tomorrow is his last game.

"We need to buy khaki shorts for *one day?*" I asked.

"Yes, and all the moms are complaining about it, too!"

"What if we just...didn't? Would he get kicked off the team? Would it go on his permanent record?"

She ignored me and wondered if we should take Kyle with us to the store. I said we should, so he can try something on. We all got into the van, but before we left, Patty told me to check my dresser to see if I already had a pair. (Kyle and I are wearing the same size now. And he's only 12.) While they waited in the van, I found two pairs in my dresser. One was a 42-inch waist. (I wear a 32-inch now.) I brought it down and showed it to Patty. She chuckled, and told me to throw it away. I also found a 34-inch pair, and Patty had Kyle try it on. It fit okay, so we didn't have to go to the store.

Wednesday, October 4, 2017

Patty said she didn't want to do anything today, but she did a bunch of housework anyway. Later, she went to see Kyle's football game at the middle school. It was his last game of the year, and it was very close, with his team losing in the last 30 seconds. Kyle didn't play in this game, though. Then, Patty got McDonald's for the kids once again. She told me this is the last time; we've been hitting the drive-through too often and now that football is over, we're going to stop. I hope she means it, but count me skeptical.

She also didn't log anything today, once again. I shouldn't be too quick to judge. I was naughty today myself, because I ate another whole bag of almond M&Ms. A very *big* bag of them. I confessed this to my boss Megan, who is also on MyFitnessPal, and she told me I needed to log it anyway. So, I did. So, I overate by 900 calories today. This is probably only going to get harder, because Halloween is coming in a few weeks. And there's going to be candy everywhere.

I've also been wondering what we are going to do about Thanksgiving next month. The last thing I want to do is plan to have a big meal. Nowadays, bountiful food has become more of a curse to avoid, rather than a blessing to celebrate. I want our family to go somewhere and do something new and different, but I don't know what just yet.

Thursday, October 5, 2017

A half hour before the alarm, Patty gently shook me awake. She was fresh out of the shower, and wearing a towel.

And nothing but a towel.

On her head.

She is uncommonly beautiful, and I have never seen her more slender. For a moment, I wasn't sure if she were real, or an erotic dream.

When she wants to, this woman can have some overwhelming sex appeal. If you ever hear me complain about anything, tell me to shut my mouth. I am the...luckiest...man...alive.

An even bigger surprise...Patty logged her food today! I wish she would log like that every day. Hell, I wish she would *wake me up* like that every day, too.

Later on, Patty had a conference at the elementary school. As she was leaving the school, one of the teachers, who had taught all three of our kids, asked Patty, "How is it that your *kids* are aging... But *you're* not? You look like you're getting younger!" Patty told me that's the best compliment she's ever gotten. She must have had a glow from this morning. Leave it to the husband to take all of the credit...

Friday, October 6, 2017

Patty did nothing today. She very *intentionally* did nothing today. At least that's what she said. When I kissed her goodbye this morning, she was wearing a t-shirt and pajama pants. She was wearing the same thing when I came home in the afternoon. She was lounging on the living room couch, watching *Dr. Phil.*

I did notice that the house seemed well-kept, and I'm sure the kids did not do a thing to help with that. So, Patty is probably underestimating the housework she did today. She often does that.

She made the two of us some riced cauliflower, but that's all she logged; that, and a small banana. Because I didn't get much sleep last night, she even let me take an afternoon nap. So, both of us allowed each other to be lazy, but just for today.

Saturday, October 7, 2017

It's another weigh-in Saturday. Bad news all around. Patty maintained at 219. I did a lot worse. I *gained* four pounds, so now I'm at 191. That's very distressing.

I went back to the MyFitnessPal app. I was wondering if resetting my strategy would do anything. I didn't expect it would, but it did. I typed in my current weight, my goal weight, how fast I wanted to lose, and my activity level. It came back with a new daily calorie number. My calorie budget dropped from 1930 to 1730 per day.

Two hundred fewer calories, every day! That's going to be hard. That really sucks.

Patty went to visit her mom at the hospital today. She says her mom is looking better, so that's encouraging. I tried my best to keep the boys from messing up the house while she was gone, but I don't think I did too good of a job.

Sunday, October 8, 2017

Patty was venting to me this morning, telling me about how frustrated she is with her mother. She complains that her mom calls her too often, even early in the morning and late at night when Patty is trying to sleep. She says that her mom forgets that she called her only ten minutes before. She doesn't think it's memory loss, instead she thinks it's an effect of her low oxygen levels. She doesn't know which is easier for her, having her mom in the hospital, or having her across the street at home. I don't know either.

I do know that Patty didn't feel like logging anything today.

Monday, October 9, 2017

Something very cool happened today. It's another milestone, not only in our weight-loss journey, but in our marriage.

While Patty was in the kitchen, I walked up to her and hugged her. That's not special; I do that all the time. But I tried something new today. I hugged her really tight. Then, I held my breath...and I grunted...and I finally did it.

After months and months of her losing weight, and months and months of me doing thousands and thousands of push-ups...it all bore fruit today. I wrapped Patty up in my arms, and I...*picked...her...up*. Right clean off the floor, several inches off the floor, and held her there, amid her sputtering and giggling and begging for me to put her down.

Never in our 22-year relationship have I ever been able to do that. But, now I can. She said it hurts her back. But she said it through the kind of satisfied smile I rarely saw from her in the past, but is more and more common now.

Tuesday, October 10, 2017

Patty had a really hard time getting Nicholas out of bed this morning. She told me to dump water on him, which is usually a sure-fire way to get him, or our other kids, out of bed. But Nicholas just allowed me to dribble water on him, and just gave me a dirty look instead of avoiding it. We're going to have to find another motivator, I guess.

Patty spent some more time up at the hospital with her mom today, and she almost didn't make it to our kids' pediatrician to pick up their prescriptions before the office closed. It was a race between her and me to see who could get there the fastest. We were coming from different sides of town, and she was a couple miles ahead of me, so she got to the doctor's office first and called me to tell me to go on home.

When I got home, I found Kyle asleep on Maverick's dog bed. I told him to get up and clean up the living room before Mom got home. He ignored me. Then I pulled off his blanket. When I walked away, he snatched the blanket off the couch where I threw it and curled back up on the dog bed. Then, I took his blanket *and* his cell phone, and he finally got the message that he had to clean up the living room. I had to inspect his work three times before I thought it was satisfactory, and Kyle complained the whole time how I was being mean. Tough luck, kid.

Wednesday, October 11, 2017

Patty made both of us breakfast today, which is unusual on a day I have to leave early. She made me an egg sandwich, which was pretty good.

Later, we had a long phone conversation. We talked about how the painting and remodeling projects cost more than we thought, and left us broke. We talked about some changes that Patty is going to make to her grocery strategy; less cereal and sweetened yogurt, and more fresh fruits for the kids as snacks.

We also talked about her weight loss journey, and about how she really should write a book, and she agreed, except she said she doesn't have any time. And she also worried about disclosing the fact that she had bariatric surgery, which is still kind of a secret. She did say that she remembered how she felt in the few weeks after surgery, when she was so tired and crampy and sore and how she really regretted the surgery for some time. She said that's the kind of thing she wants to write about, to warn others that they might feel the same way for a while, but that it's a phase they will get over.

Some days, I wonder why I'm writing all this down. Today is not one of those days.

Thursday, October 12, 2017

Patty got more groceries today. One thing about shopping for fresh food that comes in cellophane, rather than processed food that comes in boxes and cans, is that it expires sooner. So, that means that you have to buy smaller quantities, and you have to buy it more often. I know in decades past, people would "can" their food in Mason jars. Maybe that's something Patty and I should look into.

Today was a pullup day for me. I'm now able to do sets of three pullups most days I try. Today, I could *almost* do four. Between those and the pushups I do, my arms are getting developed. I can fill out the entire sleeve on most of my T-shirts. Strangers have been noticing, asking me if and where I work out. It feels good. Although I'm pleased with this accomplishment, I still want to shave another inch or two off my waist.

Friday, October 13, 2017

When Patty called me today, she said she was fighting a headache and doing laundry. She had been planning on going to a high school football game tonight to see Kyle on a float in the homecoming parade. But today, she said she wasn't really feeling up to it, and the other kids don't seem to want to go either. So she said she's thinking about having a chill day at home.

I guess chilling at home does not include logging. She logged nothing today.

Saturday, October 14, 2017

I lost seven pounds this week! I stepped on the scale with trepidation, since the shocking 191-pound reading last Saturday. When I got on today, it read 183.6 and I couldn't believe it. I had all but given up on ever getting to my goal of 180. Now, it is once again within reach. I'm thinking, given the trendline, that I'm going to gain some back next week. But, this is a good weekend anyway.

Patty does not share my enthusiasm. She only lost one pound, and is back at 219. I was gloating about my seven pounds, and now she is envious. She made me a western omelette this morning, and I had to watch her to make sure she didn't slip any extra fat into it.

We had one of my tax clients visit today, one who we hadn't seen in several months. When we opened the door for her, she took a look at us and was stunned. She called me "the incredible shrinking man," and she called Patty "the incredible shrinking woman." She knows what she is talking about, too, because she works as a personal trainer at a local gym. She and Patty talked for two hours about working out, weight control, and fad diets. Patty can now speak from a position of credibility, due to the fact she's lost 98 pounds so far.

During this conversation, we told her about MyFitnessPal, and I scolded Patty for not logging lately. She agreed, and said she needed to do better.

Later, we walked over to a neighbor's house for a neighborhood tradition called "Ice Cream for Dinner," intended for the neighborhood kids. The adults can partake as well. There were buckets of ice cream and several toppings, including syrups and chocolate chips and sprinkles and gummi bears and whatnot. Patty and I went along with Nicholas. He had some ice cream, but Patty and I did not. We only went for the conversation. Normally, I have a weakness for ice cream, but it wasn't very hard to turn it down today. I'm thinking about weighing in next weekend. I'm hoping to be very motivated this coming week.

Sunday, October 15, 2017

Patty made me some French toast today, and I was very careful about how I logged it. I remember that the cornstarch in our homemade powdered sugar has calories, so I was sure to log them. I am making a point to stick very close to my calorie budget, ignoring all the temptations in the house. Even though we don't have a lot of obviously bad stuff, like cookies or potato chips, we do have lots of seedless grapes, and some high protein ice cream. I'm trying my best to ignore all that stuff.

It was an extremely windy day at flag football today. The boys couldn't even practice, because throwing the ball is out of the question. Basically they just practiced handoffs, and ran around a lot.

Patty looks nice today, wearing a pink top and black yoga pants. I said to her, "Gosh, you're pretty." While driving to the football game, I told her, "I didn't expect this, but I married an appreciating asset."

"How is that?"

"Every month, you're getting both prettier, and healthier!"

I was hoping for a blush, or a pinch on the thigh. Instead, she just smirked and played with her iPhone.

Monday, October 16, 2017

Patty weighed in at 218 pounds this morning. That means she has lost 99 pounds since her surgery 11 months ago. She's so close to that 100-pound mark, and to celebrate, I am making plans to buy her 100 red roses, or maybe carnations, which is her favorite flower. I can't really describe in words how proud I am of her. She has made this all look easy, and of course I know it wasn't, because I'm going through this process with her. But if she wasn't there to inspire me and hold me accountable, I never could have done it myself.

Patty spent some of today taking her parents' dog to the vet, because it is having what she thinks is a liver problem. That gives me some time alone to write this journal. She hasn't logged anything so far today, so I have to pester her some. I know she had a fourth of a Wendy's chili, because she gave me the other ¾ cup.

Patty went out shopping for Halloween candy. She was debating whether to get the fun-size bars, or spring for the full-size bars. She uses full-size Hershey bars to make whatever fudge concoction she likes to make. I'm not sure exactly what she bought, because she is storing it at my mom's apartment. (We don't want our kids to find it.)

Tuesday, October 17, 2017

When we were getting out of bed this morning, Patty was talking about our trip to North Carolina next spring for our niece's wedding.

"At least we can pack more clothes than last time, because our clothes will be a lot smaller," she said. The benefits of losing weight, especially as a couple, are enormous.

For dinner, Patty made us grilled chicken and baked potatoes. Instead of sour cream, I added yogurt to mine. It tasted pretty good. Everyone else had salad with cheese and dressing, but I declined. Without the cheese and dressing, mine would have just been lettuce, which I didn't care for tonight.

Once again, no logging from Patty. I, on the other hand, haven't missed a single day. Sometimes, MyFitnessPal will congratulate me for logging a certain number of days in a row, so that's a motivation, too.

Patty's mom called here a couple of times tonight, wanting to talk to Patty. Patty was out with *my* Mom again, to pick up an online order at the store. I think her mom's voice sounds stronger than it has for a few months now. I'm hoping her oxygen level is getting back to normal.

Wednesday, October 18, 2017

Patty has been pestering me today. She reminded me that I still haven't fixed the dryer, the one in which a couple of screws fell out of the drum, and now it won't spin. I set a reminder on my phone, so that when I get home, my phone will remind me to do it.

Patty has complained about how hard it is to get our kids up and ready for school in the morning. She says she goes to bed too late, and doesn't get enough sleep. I'm thinking she ought to be able to sleep in and have the kids get *themselves* up and ready for school. She talks like that's impossible, but I know there are kids who do it every day. And they do chores when they get home, too. Now, how do we get *our* kids to do that?

Thursday, October 19, 2017

We were both tired when we got up this morning. As I was leaving, Patty asked me, "Do you need anything from the store?"

I replied, "Could you buy me some sleep?"

Patty asked Nicholas what his favorite fruit was. He replied, "Strawberries!" I would have thought his favorite fruit were grapes. He likes to dip cut strawberries in a saucer of sugar. I think that defeats the purpose, but oh well, he's a kid.

Friday, October 20, 2017

The kids were home from school today, and Patty called me all upset because Kyle had been sitting behind the chair and spilled his drink all over the new wood floor, and he had a hard time cleaning it all up. I just knew he was behind there so he could watch his iPad while snacking. I banned that practice weeks ago, but I wasn't home to enforce it.

Later on, I stopped in the store to buy a large pack of chewing gum, because of where we are going tomorrow.

Saturday, October 21, 2017

Patty weighed herself today, and she maintained at 218. That 100th pound is becoming very elusive for her. She must not be in too bad of a mood though, because I just heard her singing Carly Rae's *Call Me Maybe* down in the kitchen.

I chose not to weigh myself today. We headed south of Columbus to the town of Circleville, where they are holding their annual Circleville Pumpkin Show. This is a really big festival; I'm told it is the largest one in Ohio. They sell everything pumpkin: pumpkin funnel cakes, pumpkin waffles, deep fried pumpkin pie, pumpkin ice cream, pumpkin frozen yogurt, pumpkin doughnuts, pumpkin bread, pumpkin soup...you get the picture. Their trash cans are even orange and black, to look like pumpkins. It's an absolute orgy of pumpkin-flavored sweetness and calories.

My fear was that if I weighed myself this morning, that I knew I would not have to weigh myself for another week, and I might be more tempted to partake of all this pumpkin confectionery. So, instead, I put off my weigh-in for one more day, brought the chewing gum to the Pumpkin Show with me, and dutifully chewed gum the whole time I was there, to the amusement and eyerolls of my entire extended family that was there with us. They were eating pumpkin ice cream and pumpkin fudge. They would have bought pumpkin doughnuts, too, but they decided the line was too long. Patty even had some food there, but not pumpkin. She had beef tips, mushrooms and onions. But she ate very little of it and threw the rest away.

I don't remember the name of the song, but while we were waiting for our boys to come out of the fun house, there was a country love song coming over the speakers. Patty wrapped her arms around my shoulders and quietly, sexily, sang some of the suggestive lyrics into my ears, cradling her newly-slender body into mine. It was a love and confidence that is new for her.

Sometimes, that girl can make me melt like pumpkin fudge on the hot pavement.

Sunday, October 22, 2017

I gained a pound, to 185. All that discipline I had at the pumpkin festival yesterday was for nothing. Although, if I ate all that stuff with abandon, I'd probably have gained more. Losing seven pounds one week usually means a gain the following week anyway, given the trendline. So, I'm not doing too bad.

Patty is still stuck at 218. She is considering going back to water aerobics at the YMCA to lose that 100th pound.

Patty went to a birthday dinner last night while I was at work, and she scolded herself for the sinful "bites, licks, and tastes" she had at the steakhouse. She is not logging because she samples too many things, instead of eating a meal.

Monday, October 23, 2017

Patty has been complaining about the living room television. The reception is dropping out and pixelating. She wanted me to go outside and move the antenna that is attached to the side of the house, but I didn't have time to do it before I went to work, and I completely forgot about it after I got home. It's not at the top of my mind, because I don't watch TV.

It was raining all day today, so I didn't get to walk the dog. I was planning to do the treadmill, but it got later and later and it was time to put the kids to bed. So, I laid in bed with Patty and had all the lights off and the house quiet, so that everyone would be asleep before I went down to the treadmill. Of course, I fell asleep, too, and didn't do it. Shame on me.

Tuesday, October 24, 2017

When I got home, Patty reminded me again about the television antenna. I didn't have rain as an excuse today so, I went outside and moved the antenna around, but it didn't help. Then I plugged an indoor antenna into our TiVo box and it worked much better. I was thinking that the cord from the outside had a break in it or something. Then I noticed something else.

"Here's your problem, Patty. The antenna cable came unplugged from the wall."

She's thinking Kyle unplugged it out of spite because we made him stand in that corner a couple days ago. I'm glad it was a simple fix. Patty was threatening to order cable TV. That's an expense we don't need.

Patty sent me to Dollar General to get some Sprite for Kaitlyn, who wasn't feeling well. While I was there, I picked up some candy for the boys. Patty wasn't happy about that.

"The next time you bring in candy for the kids without telling me, I'm kicking your butt!"

"It's right here, come and kick it!"

"I can't! It's too little!"

I should tell her that I'll kick *her* butt if she doesn't log, like she didn't today. But...nah.

Wednesday, October 25, 2017

Patty went to water aerobics today at the YMCA for the first time in a couple of months. She called me afterwards, and told me that the other women there were shocked by how much more slender she looks. She said the exercise made her tired, but she was happy she did it, and she needs to do it more.

I guess Patty felt like teasing me this evening. She texted me a photo of the dinner she made: my favorite French toast, under the words "Breakfast for dinner.'" It made my mouth water. And I'm not even home. That is so unfair...

Thursday, October 26, 2017

Well, Patty was feeling amorous this morning. I don't really know why but I sure enjoyed it!

When she got dressed, Patty found an old jacket in her closet that she decided to try on. To her delight, not only was she able to get into it, it was a little too big for her. It was a black hooded fall jacket with leather panels. I told her she looks like a biker chick, and that I'm going to take her to a biker bar and we'll dance to some outlaw country.

She just ignored me, and kept admiring herself in the mirror.

Friday, October 27, 2017

Patty woke up glum this morning. She gained half a pound, even after doing the water aerobics. And she's been having a stomachache all morning.

She did get around to logging today, and ate 603 calories, even with the tummy ache. This afternoon, she seemed in a better mood. She called me to ask if I wanted to see the Maroon 5 concert here in Columbus next autumn. I answered, "Sure! I'll go see *any* concert, if it's with *you*!"

I'm thinking my happy marriage is secure for another day.

Saturday, October 28, 2017

I guess it's my turn to be glum today. I gained three pounds this week, so now I am back at 188. I have no excuses.

We went across the street to Patty's parents' house, to watch the Ohio State-Penn State football game. Patty made some salad for us. Her dad ordered a bunch of chicken wings, but I didn't eat any of them.

What a game! The Buckeyes won by one point in the final two minutes, after an amazing comeback against Penn State. We were behind the whole game, so it was very exciting. We're all in a good mood tonight.

The only thing Patty logged was one protein bar. I don't know if she had any chicken wings, but if so, she would have peeled the skin and breading off of them.

238

Sunday, October 29, 2017

We had big plans for today. We were going to clean the garage, and do the treadmill. Patty was lazy, though, by her own admission. She did do some housework and laundry, and also made me some French toast. (Yum!)

I got a few errands done. I got my brakes fixed, and I replaced the ceiling fixture in our bedroom closet. I hung Patty's new full-length mirror on our bathroom door. And I did the treadmill, which made Patty mad. She calls me selfish when I get to exercise and she doesn't. She also does that sometimes when I walk the dog. Maybe I should sit in the recliner and watch football on TV all day with a six-pack of beer and a jumbo bag of chips, right? Nah. I'll be selfish instead.

Patty didn't feel like cooking for dinner. We went grocery shopping, and then got Panda Express on the way home. I went out later and got my favorite grilled chicken wraps from Wendy's.

I logged all my food and my exercise today. I have no idea why Patty didn't.

Monday, October 30, 2017

Nicholas missed the bus this morning, so I had to drive him to his elementary school on my way to work. When a child is late, the parent has to sign him in. One of the columns on the sign-in sheet is for "reason." I wrote in, "A.M. Chaos." I'm sure they'll understand.

Nicholas is nine, and he is waffling about going out to trick-or-treat tomorrow night. The two older kids have shown no interest at all. I hope Nicky will go, because I like to walk the neighborhood on Halloween.

Tuesday, October 31, 2017

I'm depressed because our kids don't want to trick-or-treat this evening. Kaitlyn sat out in the garage with my mother passing out candy and talking to the kids and parents. I sat out with them sometimes, but Patty stayed in the living room, which surprises me. She's usually pretty outgoing and chatty. This is the first year in the eight years we've lived here that we didn't go walk the neighborhood with our kids for Halloween.

I texted my friend Charlene and told her I need grandchildren. She told me to be careful what I wished for.

Both Patty and I broke down and ate candy. We're supposed to back each other up. Maybe we were both a little down that our kids are growing up. Patty didn't log any of the candy she ate, or any of the food either. I logged my food, but I skipped logging the candy.

NOVEMBER 2017

Wednesday, November 1, 2017

*L*ast night, I didn't do my last set of pushups. I *dreamed* I did them, though. Actually, I dreamed twice about doing them. In one of the dreams, I felt like I was full of helium, and the pushups took no effort at all. That's how I knew I was dreaming.

I was planning on snoozing in bed until the kids fell asleep, then I would go in the basement and do the treadmill (to work off the candy I ate) and do my pushups. I don't know why I keep fooling myself like this. Once I'm in bed, I should know I'm going to stay there for the night.

At work today, a customer just told me I look great. Things like that make it all worth it, even though I confessed to her about the candy last night.

Patty did her water aerobics at the YMCA today, and she called me to tell me about it. She was both sore and satisfied. She also told me that Kaitlyn made the cheerleading squad at her high school for basketball season. That's not easy, either. I'm very proud of her.

Patty told me she was invited to an Amy Grant concert next month by her nephew and his wife, and she's not going to go because the seats are in the "nosebleed" section, and she'll get dizzy. I really disputed that. I remember a couple years ago when we went to see Shania Twain. Patty told me she needed earplugs, because she was afraid the loud bass in the arena would give her a migraine. When we got there and took our seats, she kicked herself for forgetting those earplugs. She had a great time, anyway. So did I.

I reminded her of that today, and told her she needs to take advantage of these special occasions to get out of her day-to-day drudgery. She defended her day-to-day drudgery, so I don't know how effective I was. But I will still urge her to go to the concert.

Thursday, November 2, 2017

This morning, Patty took Nicholas to his speech appointment. In the waiting room, there is an oversized chair that Nicky calls the "fat seat." Patty sat down in it, and had lots of room left over. Nicky nestled in beside her in the same chair. Patty texted me, "Nicky thinks it's great that we can fit in the fat seat together."

She had a very busy day today. Appointment, then taking Nicky to school. Then taking her parents' dogs to the groomer. Then more running around...I forgot everything she told me, because it was a blur. I know that I'm really lucky to have her. She's annoyed with herself for forgetting to pick up the prescriptions for Nicky and herself. She does that all the time. I'll have to set a reminder on my phone so I'll know when she is about to run out of her medicine.

It's another month, and I added a pushup to each set. Now I do 3 sets of 22 pushups, or 66, every other day. I'll keep adding one each month, until I get to 75 every other day, and then maybe 90. Or until I can't stand it anymore. Those last few pushups really do hurt. But it's an accomplished hurt.

I'm checking my phone to see if Patty logged today. She did, but only her breakfast of two eggs and shaved ham. 190 calories. I wonder why it's so hard for Patty to consistently log when it's been so crucial to *my* diet success.

Friday, November 3, 2017

Patty took time from her busy day today to begin planning a 50th anniversary party for her parents. She was reserving the hall, ordering decorations, arranging the food, and putting together a guest list. Her sisters are probably going to complain about Patty being bossy. Maybe that's because she's still got the "oldest sister syndrome." On the other hand, I predicted at the beginning of this year that she would get more assertive as she lost the weight and gained confidence. Maybe some of that is showing now.

I got another compliment today from a customer. Gosh, those never get old…

I dropped off my van at the shop to get the tires serviced. I rode my bike home, about two miles. Not really enough of a bike ride to log it as exercise, but it felt good. Patty offered to drive me there, but I didn't want to get her out of bed, and besides, I *like* riding my bike. I don't get to do it enough.

Saturday, November 4, 2017

I lost two pounds this week, down to 186. I'm just bouncing around in the 180s, and I've been doing it for months, and I may as well get used to it.

Patty ordered tickets to the Maroon 5 concert here in Columbus next September. She ordered the tickets in the handicapped section, but this time it wasn't because Patty needed the extra room. She thinks she is over that anxiety now, and she can actually enjoy herself at a concert. She got the handicapped seats in case her mom wants to come.

Sunday, November 5, 2017

I got to sleep an extra hour because of daylight saving time changing the clocks back an hour. And I got to wake up to the smell of Patty cooking breakfast.

Actually, that's not true. I spent the whole damned hour going around the house, changing the clocks. But waking up to the smell of French toast, that part is true.

Well, the volume on our living room TV has been cutting in and out, and Patty is extremely frustrated with the TV. She wants a new one. But that's expensive, so I tried to hook it up to a sound bar we had from a couple years ago, but that didn't work. So, we're off to the store to buy a new TV. I hope my credit gets approved.

Monday, November 6, 2017

That new TV is heavy. It's very big, and very, very heavy.

Years ago, I was happy with the new flat-screen TVs, because they were so much lighter and easier to handle than the big tube TVs that Patty liked to buy, and then have me carry them into the house and hoist them onto the entertainment center. I think the biggest tube TV we had was a 37-inch, and it was a real bear to pick up. A 37-inch flat-screen TV is light as a feather.

Fast forward to today, and Patty wants a 55-inch, or a 60-inch, or whatever it is. It's like the SPF number on a bottle of sunscreen; once it gets above 50 or so, does the number really matter? A big number just means, "Too damned big for one guy to pick up and mount onto the wall." This TV mounts so close to the wall, that once it's attached to the mount, there's not enough room to plug the cables into the rear panel.

So, that means I have to buy a different mount, one that swivels the TV away from the wall so I can get behind it. So, I have to log on to Amazon and buy a new mount. I told Patty, "Let's just get rid of the TV, and read books instead."

She looked at me as if I came from Mars.

Tuesday, November 7, 2017

Well, Patty actually logged something today. When I called her out on it yesterday, she said she would try to be better at it. So, today she...got better at it. She logged her breakfast of eggs and bread and peanut butter, and the apple she had for lunch. I know she had chicken and vegetables from Panda Express for dinner today, but she didn't log that. But, the day isn't over, so I won't be too hard on her. Yet.

Patty did the treadmill today, for the first time in a while. She said she was going to change it up a little, and every six minutes or so, she's going to walk faster on it. We'll see how long that strategy works. Later today, she didn't complain about being sore, like she does when she goes to water aerobics. Right now, she and Kaitlyn are at a cheer meeting at the high school, so I'm able to sit in my office and write this journal entry. The TV mount I ordered over the weekend just arrived, so, I'm just waiting for Patty to get home to help me mount the TV.

Earlier today, Patty sent me to the pediatrician's office to pick up a prescription refill for Kyle. I had to give the woman at the counter my photo ID. I handed her my driver's license, with the photo of me that was taken two-and-a-half years ago.

She looked at the license, then at me, then at the license, then at me.

Her chin dropped. She blinked at me a few times.

"What did you...*do?*"

So, there's someone else I got to tell about MyFitnessPal. And about my wife, who inspires me and holds me accountable. And lost 99 pounds herself.

Patty went to the store this evening to buy Thanksgiving stuff. She also brought home vanilla frozen yogurt and Magic Shell. All this, after I had eaten *all* my calories for today. That is just so many levels of wrong! Of course, I just had to cheat, and have a bowl of it. And I finished Patty's bowl too. Whatever the scale says this weekend, I will deserve it.

Wednesday, November 8, 2017

Wow, there is a screaming match downstairs. Our daughter missed the school bus, and Patty is telling her she did it on purpose. Patty is none too happy. First, she got me up to take her, but decided to take her to school herself. My poor wife. Our kids put her through too much.

Patty was sending out invitations to her parents' anniversary party, and she had Nicholas putting the stamps on the envelopes. While her back was turned, Nicky started sticking the leftover stamps on his face and forehead and everywhere else. Sure, it wasted money, but how can that not be adorable?

I'm checking her food log, and it is empty, once again. Come on, Patricia. I know you licked envelopes today. Couldn't you even log *that*?

Thursday, November 9, 2017

Patty put me to shame this morning. She got up, got the kids off to school, and worked out on the treadmill while I was still hitting the snooze button on my alarm.

While I was getting dressed, she came upstairs to take a shower. She was chatting with me throughout her shower, telling me about her talk with the neighbors yesterday and generally about her day. She stuck her hand out of the shower door to show me her nail polish, and I remarked that I could see the tendons in her hand. You could also see the tendons in mine, as well as the cephalic veins in my forearms. That's an indication that our body fat percentage has fallen quite a lot.

I know she wanted me to look at her nail polish, but...damn it, she opened the shower door, and she's naked in there. To hell with the nail polish. All of a sudden, I really needed a shower. I got in with her, and closed the shower door behind me.

Friday, November 10, 2017

It was very cold this morning. This year has been unusual. The summer was generally cooler than normal, while the autumn so far has been a bit warmer than normal. But today, it went back to normal. And a normal November morning is cold. I went outside to warm up my van while Patty was getting Nicholas ready for the school bus. Once I started the van, I saw the bus at our bus stop, loading children. I shouted into the house, "The bus is...here...*right now!*" Patty was still tying Nicky's shoes and getting his coat on him.

They took a little too long. As Nicky ran out of the garage, the bus pulled away.

I ordered Nicky into the back seat of my now warmed-up van and said, "Hurry! We're going to catch that school bus!"

And off we went, like Smokey and the Bandit, chasing down a school bus. Two stops later, I pulled up behind the bus and Nicky jumped out, and got in line with the other kids. That was actually kind of fun. And much better than taking him to the elementary school myself and having to sign him in.

Patty hasn't been logging her food for several days. I've got to change that. I'm going to tell her that she has to start logging every day, or I'm going to withhold sex from her.

(Yeah, right. Who the hell am *I* kidding?)

Saturday, November 11, 2017

I lost half a pound this week, so I'll keep my log at 186. I'm okay with that. I think it's the new normal. My wedding band is still loose on my finger, and my jeans are still a little loose around my waist. Patty told me I should think about getting a smaller size jean, down to a 30-inch waist, because my butt isn't filling out the size 32 jeans. I think that's a touch too small, but I got where I am by listening to my wife, so I should consider it.

Patty remains at 218, and she is frustrated. She was hoping to be below 200 by her one-year mark, which is only a few weeks away, and she knows she's not going to make that. I told her she needs to log, and she agreed. So, she promised to log her food today, and she did.

But she only logged her breakfast. She logged 328 calories for the day, as well as a half-hour on the treadmill. I know she made a bunch of pumpkin rolls for Thanksgiving today, and she told me she was snacking on those as she made them. She said it made her nauseous, and her system didn't take the sweetness very well. Over this past year, I told her that her baking days are probably over, but she resisted that claim, saying that she loved to bake things.

But today, she wasn't loving it. She agreed that I might be right.

She wasn't in *too* bad a mood today, though, because her hairdresser came to the house. I thanked the hairdresser for making Patty look beautiful.

Nicholas and I got to join in our neighborhood Nerf gun battle this afternoon. Even though it was very chilly outside, we had a couple dozen participants between the dads and the kids, with Nerf darts flying all around the neighborhood. Our neighbor Trisha even had a Wild-West soundtrack coming out of her minivan while we were shooting up the street. We had a great time.

Sunday, November 12, 2017

I guess the TV wasn't the problem. The sound was cutting out on the TV, so we assumed it was a bad TV. But the problem was in the TiVo box. A simple reboot of the TiVo fixed it.

Troubleshooting is a good habit to get into.

We did a lot of housework today. Patty cleaned out our bedroom closet, and I went through the garage and threw a lot of stuff out. Our goal is to get everything in the garage to fit along one wall, so that we can get both of our vehicles in the garage when the weather gets bad. That is going to take a lot of time to go through everything, and determine whether to keep it, sell it, or trash it. Today was a first pass. There will be many more.

Patty made me some French toast this morning, and she made herself an omelette, but she didn't eat much of it. She also got a large chili from Wendy's for dinner, but she only ate a third of that. She's been complaining that her tummy is sick, so she hasn't been eating very much.

But she's happy that she has a chance to catch up on laundry. As I write this, I can hear her singing down in the basement.

Monday, November 13, 2017

Patty had an appointment downtown this morning. The security guard at the building she went to took a long look at Patty's driver's license, and was struck by how different she looks now compared to how she appears on her license. We both may need to update our licenses.

Patty made breakfast for dinner: pancakes for the kids and French toast for herself and for me. We were out of sugar-free syrup, so we had to use regular syrup. It was so sweet as to be unappetizing, and it is sitting heavy on my stomach as I write this. I almost feel like it's a poison I have to get rid of. Later, I'm going to either walk the dog or do the treadmill. Maybe both. And I'm going to throw that syrup away.

Tuesday, November 14, 2017

This evening Patty and I went to the grocery store to pick up a few things. The place is all decked out for Thanksgiving. With turkeys, potatoes, oven bags, and cranberry sauce every-where, I'm thinking it's yet another holiday that has totally lost its mind.

Chatty Patty struck again. She found two friends in the grocery store, and talked to them for oh, I don't know, 20 minutes? Finally, I got bored and started walking around the perimeter of the store. Twice.

In the van, she looked at me in the driver's seat. She looked at my belly, and at my thighs, and said, "I feel like a big fat *blimp* next to you!"

I replied, "Nope. To *me*, you look like a jet fighter—sleek and powerful…"

Wednesday, November 15, 2017

Well, I should have had more faith in my lovely wife. She actually did log today, and she underate just a little bit. She logged 610 calories for the day. She also didn't log any exercise, although she promised to do the treadmill every day until she loses that stubborn 100th pound.

We check food labels very carefully now. We're always looking for high-protein, low-carbohydrate foods. That's why we eat a lot of eggs, cheese, and lean meats. There are other macronutrients that are important, but by default, we're only focusing on the protein and carbs.

One thing I've never been able to do is stay under my sodium budget. It's just hard to find food that has a lot of protein but not a lot of sodium. At least, any food that comes in a package with a barcode. That's the easiest food to log. Sometimes Patty will make a recipe that looks good to her, but when I ask her how many ounces of this or that in a serving, she doesn't know, so I can't log it very well. And I'm lousy at estimating. But I think of the days, not long ago, when I just ate whatever I cared to, for as long as I cared to, and didn't record it at all.

The thought of going back to those days really terrifies me.

Thursday, November 16, 2017

Patty called me today, and was telling me about starting some Christmas shopping. But first, the kids need new coats. They're growing, so that's to be expected. A couple of days ago, I tried on my old leather jacket, and it was huge on me. I must have bought it when I was at my heaviest. Not only was it too big around the waist, but the arms were inches longer than my own, and the bottom of the jacket, while it used to fall to my waist, was now well below my hips.

I took it off and threw it in the storage tub that Patty was using to collect clothes we're going to give away. She asked me if I wanted her to donate it or to sell it. I said it's years out of style, and no one is going to buy it. Then I suggested keeping it for 12-year-old Kyle, since he and I are now the same size. But, then again, it's years out of style, so...into the donate tub it goes.

Friday, November 17, 2017

SHE DID IT!!
After several weeks on her stubborn plateau, Patty weighed in this morning at 215 pounds. That means she has lost 102 pounds since her surgery. She finally crossed that 100-pound barrier that has eluded her for so long. I'm very, very proud of her.

I posted a before-and-after photo of the two of us on Facebook today, and wrote a congratulatory note to Patty on the post. The comments and likes flooded in by the dozens and dozens. Patty called me, and when I answered, she said, "You're too much."

"You don't have to post *everything*," she told me. But this wasn't just everything. This was a big, hairy deal. This was an important milestone on her journey. I wanted to celebrate it. And while she dismissed the post with her casual nonchalance, I know, deep within her, she was beaming like a little girl.

Christopher White is with **Patricia White**.

Nov 17, 2017 at 12:57 PM · 🌐

Warmest congratulations to my wife, **Patricia White**...

As of this morning, Patty has logged a weight loss of ONE HUNDRED FREAKING POUNDS!!!

(And not only that--she inspired ME to do the same 🙂)
❤️ ❤️

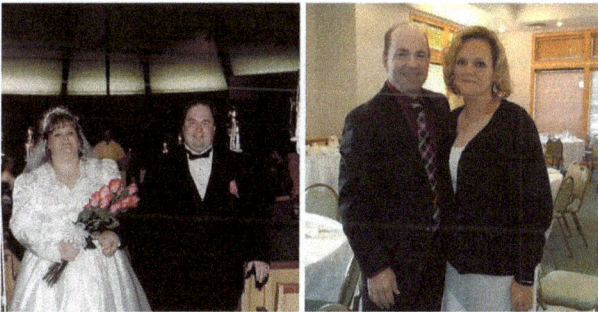

👍 Like   💬 Comment   ↗ Share

👍❤️ **Charlene and 79 others**

I was hoping to order her a bouquet of 100 flowers today, but work got too busy and I didn't get a chance. I'll be doing it soon. I'm excited for her. Today, I'm very glad I traveled down this road with her. I've never felt closer to my wife. So, I'm getting off this laptop, and going upstairs to cuddle with her. Right now.

Saturday, November 18, 2017

Patty lost yet another pound today, so she is down to 214. She still complains about the sagging skin on her arms, and around her tummy. I probably don't help, because when I hug her from behind, I like to play with that loose skin around her belly, and she gets mad at me. I tell her I only do that because she will lose it eventually, but she still is very self-conscious about it.

We have a very messy, cluttered garage and we spent an hour or so today going through it, boxing stuff up to take to the dump, and marking stuff we hope we can sell. My goal is to clear enough space in our two-car garage to actually park two cars in it. Her goal is to set up a couple of tables in the garage for Thanksgiving next week. She said we could have as many as 30 people visit us for Thanksgiving dinner, and we don't have room in the house for all of them.

I was hoping we could skip the whole "food culture" aspect of Thanksgiving and instead go on a weekend trip. But, she said she wanted to be traditional, at least for this year. Although, during the last couple of days of planning and shopping and advance preparation, she is getting a little fed up with Thanksgiving herself. Next year, I'm going to remind her of that.

Patty has been complaining of being very tired. After we worked in the garage for a while, we both gave up and watched the Ohio State-Illinois game. It was not a very exciting game. Patty was curled up in a blanket on the couch, and kept drifting off. I went upstairs, and took a half-hour nap myself. Today was cold and rainy, and a good day for a nap.

I also weighed myself today, and for the third week in a row, I maintained at 186 pounds. It seems my body has put itself into maintenance mode, without my direction. Now, I'm less focused on losing weight and more focused on avoiding weight gain.

Sunday, November 19, 2017

We had our niece and nephew stay the night last night, and Patty made pancakes for them and French toast for herself and me this morning. Then, she took Kaitlyn to the high school to get cheerleading team pictures, while the boys and I brought boxes of extra flooring from the garage downstairs to the basement.

When Patty got home, she looked through more stuff we're cleaning out of the garage, and she found a pink Columbia jacket. She just had to try it on. It was Kaitlyn's jacket, and it fit Patty. It fit well. She's keeping it.

Kyle keeps getting into the Thanksgiving food (Hawaiian buns are his favorite now) and we have to lock up the food in the locked cabinet in the garage and in Patty's locked van.

She is more resolute now about this being the last Thanksgiving that our family will celebrate with a big meal. I've been suggesting we go for a weekend trip to Canada (where they don't have Thanksgiving, or at least not at the same time the U.S. does); either to Niagara Falls or to the Windsor, Ontario area. Then, Patty mentioned wanting to go to Dollywood in Tennessee that weekend. Since we both lost weight, we like the thought of travelling to new places. But the two of us want to go in different directions...

Monday, November 20, 2017

Patty's posture is better now. She stands up straight, and doesn't hold onto a table or a counter or a chair or anything like she used to. She also crosses her legs when she sits on the couch. She told me it used to be she was not able to do that and she said again that she feels better going to concerts or to a theater. Maybe that's a hint?

Tuesday, November 21, 2017

Patty is anxious about going to her doctor next week for her one-year anniversary appointment. She hasn't lost as much weight as she wanted to. She tried a protein bar today that was new; she said it had 30 grams of protein but it had eight grams of sugar which was too much. She says eating anything sweet makes her stomach upset.

Wednesday, November 22, 2017

More and more Thanksgiving preparation today. We're cleaning out the garage because we need to put some tables full of food out there, because there won't be enough room in the house.

Patty is making deviled eggs, and double layer pumpkin pie, and turkey breast, and ham, and I forget everything she told me, but it's more than plenty.

Patty received the ring today that she ordered a couple days ago. She hasn't been wearing her wedding ring because it's too loose on her. And since she hasn't really had time to go and get a new ring and set the diamond in it, she just ordered a costume ring for a few dollars. She likes the look of it enough that she sent a picture to me.

Thursday, November 23, 2017

It's a full-on stress test on Patty this Thanksgiving Day. She's mashing potatoes and slicing ham and turkey, and shouting orders to the boys and me, to pick up the messy house and get chairs and tables arranged. I'm getting cans of food from the pantry and garage as she calls for it, and throwing away bags of trash and empty cans as she generates them. I already can't wait until next year, when she promises to skip the whole Thanksgiving Dinner thing and take ourselves and our kids on a trip somewhere instead.

I cautioned her not to use the garbage disposal today. "Never, ever use the garbage disposal on Thanksgiving. You'll clog it up, and plumbers are expensive today. Just use a bucket instead."

She found out she bought a cajun turkey, instead of a regular turkey. She loudly proclaimed, "I'm such an idiot!"

"I'm *glad* you're an idiot. Otherwise, you wouldn't have married *me*."

That garnered me a smile and a kitchen kiss.

The dinner went really well. We had a couple dozen people here, and we were able to seat them all somehow. I ate turkey, noodles, and mashed potatoes, and had a range of desserts: double-layer pumpkin pie, pumpkin bar, fudge, and seedless grapes. And I didn't log any of it. (I *did* log the pullups I did, though.)

There was plenty of food left over, and thankfully, our visitors took a lot of it with them. Patty did a lot of cleaning up, but she didn't complain too much. I helped her as much as I could, and resisted the temptation to go take a nap. Patty had thought about going Black Friday shopping tonight, but at the end of the night, she was too tired and went to bed before the boys and I did. Kaitlyn is still out shopping with her aunt and cousins, so I'm waiting up for her.

While waiting, I opened MyFitnessPal and did a search for "Thanksgiving." There was an entry, a "Thanksgiving meal" for 1200 calories. I logged two of those meals. That might just cover it.

Friday, November 24, 2017

We both slept late, which was welcome. Patty got up first, and made breakfast and cleaned the house. When I got up, she tasked me with unpacking the Christmas tree and the storage tub full of ornaments and trimming.

Before we could put up the tree, we had to move the living room furniture. Patty told me the most delightful thing I've heard in months: she said we're giving the recliner to my mom! *Finally!* I'm about to be rid of that damned recliner, that I've never sat on, and that I never wanted in the first place.

So, I got Kyle off of his Xbox and he and I wrestled the recliner out through the garage, into my van, and into my mom's apartment. After I got home, I checked the fridge for a snack, and saw a leftover double-layer pumpkin pie. It is one of Patty's legendary specialties, and it has always been irresistible.

However, I resisted. I didn't touch any of it. Patty didn't eat any of it, either. I sense the beginning of a standoff, each of us trying to out-resist the other, just daring the other to eat that wonderful pie.

I think I have an unfair advantage, simply because I'm writing about it. But, as of yet, Patty doesn't know that.

Saturday, November 25, 2017

I gained four pounds this week. I'm not too upset about that, since it was not unexpected. Patty also gained four pounds. She is beside herself disappointed. She's going on and on about how her doctor is going to hate her when she sees him in four days.

We went across the street to her parents' house to make brunch. Patty made us all some Western-style omelettes, and her Aunt Nancy helped make some fruit salad. So, that was our brunch. Patty often fills her plate with the stuff she makes, and then can only eat about a third of it. Then she offers it to me, and I won't eat it, because I already ate what she gave me and I logged it. I'm not going to fall for that anymore.

Brunch was not the main reason we went across the street, though. We went there to watch the game. Rather, "*The Game*". The greatest rivalry in all of sport. Carmen Ohio, Gold Pants, and O-H-I-O in the Big House. Ohio State vs. Michigan. It was a great game this year. Michigan jumped out to a 14-0 lead in the first quarter. Then the Buckeyes clawed their way back, and dominated the fourth quarter. Ohio State won the game 31-20. It's party time here in Columbus!

Sunday, November 26, 2017

I didn't have French toast yesterday because we didn't have the high-protein bread Patty uses to make it. I brought some home last night, so Patty was able to make it this morning for me. Our weekends are not complete without it.

Patty didn't feel good most of the day today. After we hung up some laundry, she sat down on the couch and I sat with her. I cuddled with her and rubbed her shoulders. I started kissing her and coaxing her to the bedroom, but she refused, citing her tummy ache. (Which I knew would happen. But I haven't been initiating sex as much as she has, and I didn't want her to think I'm uninterested.) I did tell her how much better it is to cuddle with her now that I can fit my arms all the way around her, and still be able to touch my elbows.

She made taco cups for dinner. Those are made with wonton wraps pushed into a muffin pan, and baked with lean ground beef, green onions and sour cream. I ate five of them and they were only 250 calories or so. Later, I did the treadmill for almost an hour, and did my pushups too. Patty commented that she created a monster in me, and that she wished she had the energy to do the exercises I do.

Monday, November 27, 2017

I woke up very sore. Patty says it's because of all the pushups I do, but I've been doing them for months, and they don't make me as sore as I was today (at least not anymore). I was also tired. I got up twice overnight because I caught Nicholas under his blanket playing a game on his iPad. I finally had to take it from him and put it under my pillow.

It was a busy day at work, and Patty had a busy day also. Sometimes when I come home late, Patty doesn't want to cook, so she sends me to pick up food somewhere. Tonight, it was Chick-Fil-A. She got a market salad, and I got grilled chicken cool wraps. The kids got sandwiches and fries. I splurged on a cookies and cream milkshake, and so I'm 340 calories over budget today. I'm going to have to do the treadmill before bed.

We visited our nephew's new house this evening. His appliances looked familiar. Then I remembered Patty and I gave our old appliances to him and his wife when we got the new ones a few months ago. It's nice to see they still worked.

On the way home, I was going through an intersection and looking out the passenger window past Patty. She smiled at me and said, "I'll bet it's easier to look around me now." I agreed with her, even though I don't remember it being difficult to look around her even *before* she lost the weight. But, if it makes her feel better, I'll go with it.

Tuesday, November 28, 2017

Patty has logged many accomplishments this year. Today, she added another one. She saved a life.

She was at lunch at a Bob Evans restaurant with her Aunt Nancy. Another guest at the restaurant was choking and turning blue, and Patty sprung into action and began a Heimlich maneuver on the woman. She was helped by another guest, and together they got the food out of the woman's windpipe, and she started breathing again. If it were up to me, she would get a medal.

She brought home Wendy's today, and I ate one chicken wrap and a chocolate frosty for dinner. Then I took Maverick for a walk. It was a brisk walk, because Maverick was energetic this evening. I hope it was enough to walk off that frosty.

Patty ate a little bit of chili, but I think that's it. She sees her doctor in the morning for her one-year surgery anniversary, and she is dreading the scale.

Wednesday, November 29, 2017

Today is the one-year anniversary of Patty's surgery. She lost 103 pounds, before putting four pounds back on because of

Thanksgiving week. She went to see her surgeon today, and he seemed very happy with a weight loss of 99 pounds. Patty is not very happy about it, though. She thought the surgeon would be disappointed, but he wasn't.

Patty has also gone a whole year without having to go to the emergency room due to back pain. She used to have to go every few months, and get a pain shot in her lower back. But, since the surgery, she hasn't gone once. And, avoiding all that pain, time, inconvenience, and *expense*...That's a very big accomplishment.

After work, I stopped by the pharmacy to pick up my own prescription. The pharmacist asked for my birthdate, and I told him. From behind me came an astonished, 'Nuh-uhhh!" I glanced behind me, and the woman there looked stunned. Then she craned her neck to look at me more closely.

She then told the pharmacist, half-jokingly, "You should check his ID. I don't believe that birthdate!"

(So much for HIPAA compliance, I suppose.)

I smiled, and pulled out my driver's license. I didn't give it to the pharmacist, but showed it to the woman instead. The license is over two years old, back when I was still nearly 300 pounds. The woman smiled, returned the license, and gave me a high-five. "That's incredible. Wow!"

This, from a total stranger.

You've heard of Cloud Nine? Yeah, that's the one. It's down there, a couple clouds below me right now.

Thursday, November 30, 2017

I've noticed that I haven't been food-stalking Patty. Meaning that, I haven't been checking the MyFitnessPal app to see what she has been logging, or if she has been logging at all.

Since she reached the 100-pound weight-loss milestone, and since she essentially eats similar things every day, it was becoming...uninteresting.

Today, she admitted that she has not been logging lately, and she feels that she has been backsliding. She met another bariatric patient at her surgeon's office, and I guess this other patient and Patty are going to compete and collude to lose another 20 pounds each over the next four months.

So, Patty began logging again today. I'm glad that she found a new source of motivation. I'm a little bewildered, though, that *I* couldn't continue to be her source of motivation. I told her I would lose 20 more pounds along with her.

She shouted, "*No!* You're too skinny *already!*" When she's in the room while I'm doing my pushups, she just rolls her eyes and tells me I've gone overboard. Then she shouts out random numbers, so I lose count. Then she tells the dog to lick me and make me laugh, so I'll have to stop. It's like she's given up trying to keep up with me. Maybe I should back off, or slow down a little?

Hell, no. This kind of hurt feels too good.

DECEMBER 2017

Friday, December 1, 2017

I've beaten a few food addictions on this journey of ours. I used to be able to eat a pound or two of chocolate covered raisins, but I gave that up when I started reading nutrition labels. My craving for ice cream is well-known, and I try to keep it out of the house. Of course, the typical drive-through food of fried chicken sandwiches and French fries have been erased from my routine long, long ago.

But not all my addictions are gone. My current problem is red, seedless grapes. Patty brings them home every week, and I can't stop eating them. They're not a bad food to eat, but it's the one food where portion control is impossible for me. If I eat a nine-ounce cup full of them, I'm not satisfied and I have to have more. Then I eat the whole three-pound bag. That's what I did today. I used to be able to chew gum to take my mind off the grapes, but I didn't have any gum today. So, I'm still battling with food cravings, even after losing a hundred pounds.

Patty went to the high school basketball game where Kaitlyn is cheering. I think she got McDonalds on the way home, because I saw the bag of trash when I got home from work. Patty has been pestering me to put up outside Christmas lights on the house, which I hate, and I'm trying to avoid doing that. She might hire someone else to do it. I don't really want to spend the money, but I certainly don't want to do it myself.

Saturday, December 2, 2017

It was a good week for the both of us. Patty lost two pounds of the four she gained last week, so she is at 216. I lost the four I gained from Thanksgiving, so I'm back at 186. I also added another pushup to each set, so I'm doing 23 per set, three sets every other day. My goal is to do three sets of 25, every other day. I'll get there in February.

I went to the bank this afternoon to cash a check, and when I handed my license to the teller, her jaw dropped. So, I got to show the before and after pictures of Patty and me that I keep on my phone for such occasions. The teller is on a weight-loss journey herself, and we talked about how we survived Thanksgiving week. Getting noticed like that makes me feel good. Of course, when I told Patty about it, I got her typical response...a snort and an eye roll.

Patty did some Christmas shopping today, and then called me in a panic, saying she thinks her van has been stolen. She couldn't find it. She came out the door at the store, couldn't find the van, then hit her keyfob's panic button to make the horn sound, but heard nothing. I was home at the time, and I went searching for our spare key. If I couldn't find the spare key, then I'd know it was in the van and maybe that's how it was stolen. But, the spare key was right where I keep it.

Just then, Patty called back and said she was mistaken. The store she went to had two entrances, and she had inadvertently went out the wrong one, and that's why she couldn't find her van. She said that was a very rattling feeling for her. It was for me, too.

Sunday, December 3, 2017

Patty did a little Christmas shopping today, and she brought home some ice cream for the kids. I had a bowl of it, because I had done the treadmill and had enough calories for it. Even Patty had a little bit, but she said it made her nauseous.

She asked me if it's okay to throw up. Huh?

It was actually a good question. She hasn't thrown up since her surgery over a year ago. She's not even sure she *can*, because her stomach is so small. Of course, I have no idea if she can or not. I told her to ask her bariatric Facebook group.

Thankfully, she didn't throw up.

Monday, December 4, 2017

Patty is still sick. The ill feeling has traveled from her stomach to the muscles in her head, neck, shoulders, and back. So, when I came home, I was expecting the house to be a little messy.

Instead, it was immaculate. It even *smelled* good. She had vacuumed, and mopped, and was downstairs doing laundry when I found her. I told her how great everything looked, and rubbed her back and shoulders. She gave me a basket to bring up, full of sheets and pillowcases for our bed. Together, we dressed the bed, and then she sent me to the store for Christmas lights and extension cords for the outside of the house. Meanwhile, she relaxed and watched *The Flash* on TV with Nicholas.

Sometimes, I think she gets more done when she is sick than when she is well. I've been whining to her about wanting sex, but I backed off the last couple days because she didn't feel good. But, she surprised me tonight when we went to bed. Should I feel guilty? Or exhilarated? I'll have to sleep on that.

Tuesday, December 5, 2017

Patty's stomach is feeling better, but she is still sore, and now she has lost her voice, too. That makes it hard to hear her on the phone. She was diagnosed with a sinus infection. Our two older kids were also sick, so she kept them home today. She went to drop off her antibiotic prescription, and wanted to wait for it to be filled before going home, but the kids were fighting in the van and giving Patty such a headache, that she went home without the medicine and asked me to pick it up on the way home, which I did.

She made us a very winter-friendly dinner tonight. Tomato soup, chicken noodle soup, and grilled cheese sandwiches. She added turkey and onion to my sandwich. We haven't had that kind of meal for a while, and it was very good on a cold evening. But at 976 calories, it wasn't very diet-friendly.

I forgot to do my pullups before going to work this morning, so I'm going to try to do double this evening. (That's a joke.)

Wednesday, December 6, 2017

I received several photos of Patty via text, but not from Patty. They were from Kaitlyn. These were photos of Patty as a schoolgirl, and some as a baby and as a toddler. It is striking how much they looked like Kaitlyn. I suspect Patty pulled out the box of old photos to find some "before" pictures of herself, but the ones that impressed Kaitlyn the most were the photos of Patty as a child, before she had weight problems.

It is much colder outside this week. Well below freezing. I am now reminded how a large drop in weight can leave you susceptible to cold weather. Our electric blanket from last year had already worn out, so we bought another one. On nights like this, I'm very glad we did.

Thursday, December 7, 2017

While I was at work, Patty took the kids to the mall to do some Christmas shopping. She said she may never do that again. She complained about the crowds and the lines. I didn't think that was such a big deal anymore in our modern, online shopping world, but I guess I was wrong. Patty got some tree ornaments made with our kids' names on them and themed with their favorite activities. She sent me photos of the ornaments, and they were very cute.

Today was a pullup day for me. I can consistently do four pullups in a set, and occasionally I can do a fifth one. While I was out driving today on the freeway, I went under a pedestrian overpass. The overpass was fenced in with a wraparound fence, and there were crossbars above the walkway that were connecting the fencing together. As I drove beneath, I saw a man doing pullups, using one of the crossbars as his pullup bar.

I'm with you, brother, I'm with you…

Friday, December 8, 2017

Despite her sinus infection, Patty spent some serious time in the kitchen today, making pans of lasagna and dessert, and

I don't know what all, for her parents' 50th anniversary party tomorrow. Her Aunt Nancy spent much of the day here with her, and Patty loves those visits.

Now, Patty just prepared Thanksgiving dinner two weeks ago, and she is probably going to contribute to Christmas dinner a couple weeks from now. I had thought that a year after the surgery, Patty would be finished with the holiday baking marathons. Silly me.

Kaitlyn has been texting me more of her baby pictures that she's been discovering in our box of family photos. While I remember the pictures, they are completely new to her. She also found a few photos of *me*, while I was holding her or reading a book to her as a baby. I remember these pictures too, but they were shocking to see. I've been getting used to seeing myself at my current weight, so when I look at these old photos of my 300-pound self, they are eye-popping. Kaitlyn summed it up best in her caption:

"Wow, Dad, you were fat!"

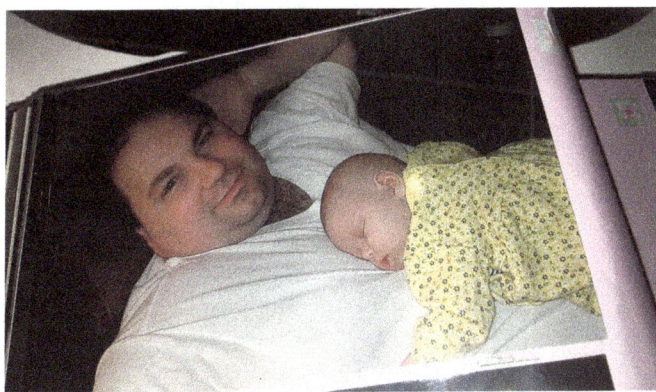

Kaitlyn: "Wow, Dad, you were fat!"

Saturday, December 9, 2017

Tonight was the big 50th anniversary party for Patty's parents, and the turnout was good, even in the snow. Patty looked beautiful in a black skirt and red sweater, but her knee-high leather boots were way too big for her thinner legs. It was funny to watch her zip up her boots and *still* be able to put both hands between the leather and her leg, with room to spare. She called it a "non-scale victory." I called it "an excuse for Patty to buy some new boots."

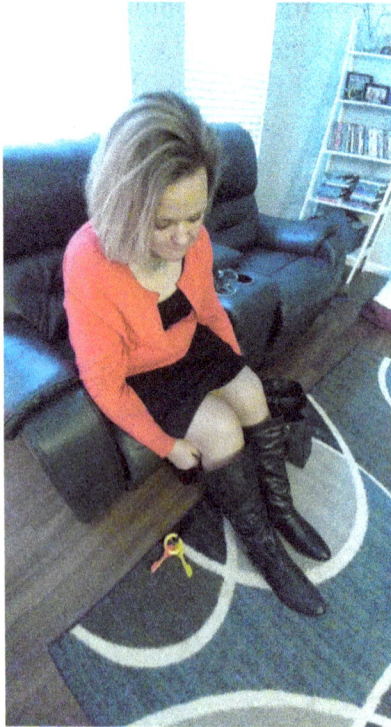

Patty tries on the leather boots that
used to be too small for her. December 2017.

I'm supposed to be happy that we don't buy so much food. That we don't have to pay for the extra-large clothes. That we don't seek nearly as much medical care. Okay, I *am* happy. But clothes are still expensive. And women's clothes are *more* expensive. And when a woman feels newly beautiful, well...her closet has needs, and my wallet is in peril.

I gained three pounds this week. Red grapes, mostly, but also something Patty calls "Christmas Crack", which is broken-up toffee brittle covered with chocolate and other stuff and is tasty enough not to log in your app. I really have to stop that.

Sunday, December 10, 2017

I must have caught something at the party last night. I couldn't sleep well at all. My sinuses were persistently clogged, and would not clear. I have a very hard time sleeping when I have to breathe through my mouth. I sought relief from a bottle of expired nose drops in the back of my nightstand drawer, but it was only effective for an hour or so.

I did my morning pushups, and I learned that pushups are hard to do when you can't breathe and your muscles are already sore. When I complained to Patty about it, she demanded I go to urgent care and get seen. Great, more expense and inconvenience. I resisted, and she persisted. I went. It was a sinus infection. Antibiotics and cough syrup for me. I hope I sleep better tonight.

We ate better today. Patty's French toast for breakfast (I have actually saved a meal in MyFitnessPal called "Patty's French Toast," and it's 655 calories for three slices), no lunch, and salad and air-fried chicken for dinner. That, and sleeping off our sinus infections on the couch by the fire.

Monday, December 11, 2017

I picked up my antibiotics from the pharmacy yesterday, after the urgent care visit. They had to order the cough syrup, so I picked that up today. The pharmacy tech asked for my driver's license, and did a double take. (Yep, the license thing again.) I looked at it myself, at my nearly 300 pounds, and it looks ghastly. Think of your worst driver's license photo, and then add a hundred pounds to it. Yeah, that bad. I like how I look now much better.

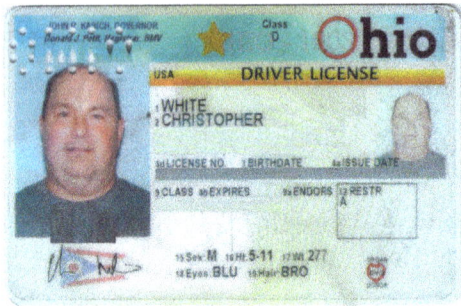

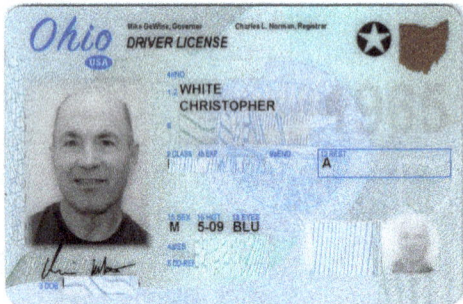

We went to a Bob Evans restaurant this evening for a birthday dinner for Nicholas, who turns 10 tomorrow. This restaurant is known for its comfort food, and it was really tough to find something to eat that was not chock-full of calories. I opted for the Chicken Cranberry Pecan salad with no dressing. Patty got a grilled chicken something, and she only ate a third of it. Then it was time to pass around the cupcakes. I refused mine, to the poking derision of my family. Hey, I already over-ate today, and I'm not going to eat a cupcake. To shut them up, I did eat the icing off of one.

After dinner, Patty and Kaitlyn went to the hospital to see the new baby, Luna. It was our nephew's daughter, who (according to Google) is our grandniece. I didn't go, because I still had sniffles, and I had stuff to do at home anyway. I helped Nicholas set up the new videogame he got for his birthday, and then I did stuff in my home office, like writing this journal entry.

Tuesday, December 12, 2017

Nicholas turns 10 years old today. It must be hard for a kid to have his birthday so close to Christmas. We have two nephews in that same boat. One of them, Dylan, has his birthday on Christmas Eve, the poor guy.

Patty is still sick from her sinus infection, although mine is pretty well gone after two days. She says she is jealous of me. She went to her family doctor today for a scheduled visit, and she weighed in at 210. She says she doesn't trust the doctor's scales, because she weighed 214 just a couple days ago. I asked if she threw up, and she said no. But she is probably dehydrated because she is sick, so that might be it. Or, maybe the scale *is* off.

She spent much of this evening on the couch under a blanket. She had me make mac and cheese for the kids, and started talking me through the process. I cut her off, reminding her that I could read the directions on the box. After it was done, she wanted a bite. She said it was remarkably good, seeing that it was made by a rank amateur. I'll take that as a compliment. And all three kids actually ate their dinner, which doesn't always happen even when *she* makes it. So there!

Wednesday, December 13, 2017

Patty is still complaining about being tired today, even though she is not complaining about the sinuses anymore. She is frustrated that even after losing over 100 pounds, she does not feel the energy she was hoping to feel. It's mid-December, and there is very little daylight this time of year. It's cold and windy, and that can lull the body into a desire to hibernate. Patty said she wishes I could come home and we could burrow under some blankets and cuddle.

I wish that too.

I'm struggling with my diet discipline in the face of Christmas candy and cookies everywhere I go. I ate a chocolate covered cherry today, and a handful of homemade hard-tack candy. I declined the chocolate-chip cookies I was offered, but I took a handful of the chocolate chips themselves. I wish this month of temptation would get over with, so I can enjoy a return to calorie sanity.

Thursday, December 14, 2017

Before I left for work this morning, Patty wanted me to watch a clip of a *Good Morning America* segment she recorded from last week. It was about Lexi and Danny Reed, an Indiana couple that lost 400 pounds together, and had documented their journey on Instagram under the name "fatgirlfedup."

Patty told me, "We should have done that, too!"

I thought about this (still secret) journal, and smiled to myself.

Patty wore a pink top and black pants, and I thought she looked beautiful. She was putting on her coat, and she commented that her mother had said that she was proud of her.

She *ought* to be proud; she has a beautiful, accomplished daughter.

I went to a warehouse dock this morning, and when the woman there opened the door she turned and called for one of the other women in the office. She yelled, "There's a cute guy at the dock!" Instinctively, I glanced around me.

There was no one at the dock...but me. I'm really not used to that.

Friday, December 15, 2017

Patty is running around town in a panic because she said she doesn't have Christmas shopping done yet, and it's getting hard to find the things she wants. I figured she was doing it all online, but I guess she was trying to look for better deals in the stores.

I thought it was a lousy idea. But, I remain very grateful that she takes those burdens off of me.

I worked outside all day, and it was cold and windy. My muscles are cold, tired, and sore. I forgot to do my pullups this morning, so I did them when I got home. I could only do three. But I'm glad I tried. If I blow it off one day, the next days will be all the easier to forget them.

Patty got into the baking mood tonight, and she texted me a list of baking needs for me to buy before I came home. She needed peanuts, vanilla bark, peanut butter chips, toffee chips, and whipping cream. I have no idea what she plans to make, but she's putting thousands of calories into it.

Saturday, December 16, 2017

Patty spent the day baking, and sending me to the store on emergency runs for sweet cream butter and heavy whipping cream. She has our nieces Brittany and Sarah over, and I'm told that the kitchen smells wonderful, but I'm trying to stay out of it. I think this is an echo of a past life, and I hope that going forward, we quit centering our holidays around food, and instead find some experiences to share.

Sunday, December 17, 2017

I have learned that Patty has been using all those ingredients to make...fudge. But not any kind of fudge. I've come to call it "Felony Fudge," because it's so good it should be a crime. Nothing about it is healthy, and I ate too much of it. I weighed myself yesterday and I have gained a pound, up to 190. I fear I won't be able to maintain until Christmas is over next week.

Patty has been complaining that she doesn't have any energy. That surprises her, because she's lost a hundred pounds and she should feel like a dynamo. She really looks pretty and I tell her that all the time. Of course, I've told her that all throughout our marriage, so she's immune to it now.

Maybe she's been sampling too much of her Christmas baking treats. I have learned that when I eat too much sugar now, it saps *my* energy, too.

Monday, December 18, 2017

Today was a pushup day, and when I was doing my afternoon set, Patty was encouraging the dog to lick me. Maverick wouldn't do it. Undeterred, Patty walked up to me, stooped down and tickled me. That was so mean! You can't get the same benefit when you break up your pushups. Does she not know that? Does she not care?

Patty made meat loaf and mashed potatoes tonight for dinner. Tomorrow she will make taco cups, or so she says. This month is not the healthiest, and we've both got to get with the program.

Tuesday, December 19, 2017

Patty was too exhausted to make taco cups. Instead, she sent me to McDonald's. She says her new year resolution is to stop feeding fast food to the kids, although she has said that before. It costs too much and it's not good for them. Of course, that means more work for herself. I think our kids are old enough to help with the cooking and cleaning.

For that matter, I think I'm old enough to help, too, right? Excuse me while I empty the dishwasher.

Wednesday, December 20, 2017

We had a little pillow talk before going to sleep tonight. Patty was reveling in her "non-scale victories." She went shopping at Kohl's and she could try on clothes and admire herself. She says everything she tried on looked good, and she wanted it all. That is not an experience she's ever had before. She tries on rings and bracelets and they all fit. It was a confidence-building day for her. Lucky for me, she didn't buy very much. But she left the store in a good mood anyway.

And I'm very proud of her. I'm glad she can enjoy herself like that.

Thursday, December 21, 2017

Patty is really tired today. She has a niece and a nephew staying the night, and they have our own kids ramped up, as well. So, Patty has a noisy house a few days before Christmas, and it is sapping her energy. I'm working more than expected today, so I'm not home to help her and I wish I were. Chores are starting to pile up and neither of us has the energy to do them. First day of winter. Not fun.

Friday, December 22, 2017

One criticism I've had about Patty and her weight issues has been her camera shyness. We started having kids 14 years ago, and Patty has never wanted to appear in any photos with them, or with me. Today she agreed with me, and she said she's not going to rob her children of any more memories and she's going to appear in lots of pictures now that she feels much more comfortable in front of a camera. That made my heart sing.

Patty and I each got a Facebook message today from my friend Angie from high school. She said she and her husband are going on a mission to get healthy, and she wanted Patty and me to tell her how we managed to do it. So, now people are starting to look to *us* to learn how to lose weight. What a reversal of fortune.

Saturday, December 23, 2017

The holiday hex is in full swing. I gained another three pounds this week, so I'm at 193. That's eleven pounds more than my lowest weight. I've been eating too much of Patty's Felony Fudge, and it's threatening my achievements.. This has got to stop.

Patty gave me a bunch of her Christmas sweets and told me to take them to work. Not so much to be nice, but to get them the heck out of the house. Neither of us need the temptation. So for the 20-minute drive to work, I carried a great big bowl of Felony Fudge and cookies and other goodies. In years past I would eat half of the bowl, or more, all by myself. But this time I just put the container in the back seat and didn't touch it. In fact, I didn't even *think* about it. That was quite a change.

When I got to work, my boss Megan told me that she has gained 13 pounds since *her* lowest weight point. We were consoling each other while both eating a piece of fudge. She said she can't wait until Christmas is over, and I agree.

Sunday, December 24, 2017

Patty and I were both in a good mood this morning. Well, more like this afternoon, because we went to bed around 5 a.m. and got up a little after noon. We sent the kids to take the dog outside, and then Patty and I showered together (it's delightful how easily the two of us fit in our small shower). Even though it's a busy Christmas Eve and we've got a lot to do, we took a little time and made a little love.

Patty's been telling me how she needs to be a better wife for me. I think she's ridiculous. She's the *best* thing to happen to me since birth!

We're renting that same VFW hall for our extended family Christmas gathering tonight. It's getting to be a big family, with a nephew newly married and another nephew becoming a dad. Just keeping track of everything is a big job, and it's no wonder Patty is tired all the time. She is looking lovely though; even Nicholas told her she's beautiful today. Patty tries to hide her glow, but she can't. She's wearing a grateful grin that just can't be erased, nor should it be. I cannot contain my pride and affection for her.

Patty and Kaitlyn are planning a trip to visit Patty's cousin in Rhode Island next month. She was talking to her Aunt Nancy, who is going on the trip as well. Patty said today (with a certain pride) that she'll be able to fit all her clothes for the weekend in a small carry-on bag, because she is so much smaller now. Another non-scale victory.

During the Christmas party tonight, it was about time to do my pushups. So, I challenged my nephew Dylan to do them with me. (Dylan was up to the challenge, having recently spent some time in the US Army.) We found a spot on the floor and got started, to the surprise and hollers of the crowd. He finished first, but not by much. Not too bad a performance for me, a man twice Dylan's age.

Monday, December 25, 2017

I usually look forward to Christmas Day as a relaxing break from all the pre-holiday gatherings we typically have. But we had a pretty big one here at the house today. We had about 15 people visit us, which took some preparation and cleanup all by itself.

My mom's car would not start, so I was called out to go and pick her up. On the way, Patty called me in a panic saying she did not have enough cinnamon to make her homemade cinnamon rolls. So I went to a gas station to see if I could find some cinnamon, and while I was there she called back to say never mind, she had found some.

And we had another round of not the healthiest food, with sausage gravy and biscuits and more Christmas candy. My niece's fiancé showed off his professional-grade video drone, which was really cool. I got into a political argument with some of the older members of the family, which was also pretty cool. And we both got to show some "before and after" pictures of ourselves. There is one where I look absolutely atrocious! I don't mind showing *that* one off now...

After I returned from taking my mom back home, I asked Patty if she would divorce me if I went straight to bed, because I was pretty tired. She didn't answer; she just gave me a dirty look. She was cleaning the kitchen and loading the dishwasher, and she sent me to hook up the DVD player in our bedroom so we could all go to bed and watch a movie.

Tuesday, December 26, 2017

Wow, last night was awful for me. We went to bed early because we were both very tired, and decided to clean the house later today. I went to bed and started to feel bloated, and then nauseous. I had chills and sore muscles, and even having the electric blanket on high didn't help. After a couple of hours, the nausea got the better of me, and I hurried into the bathroom to throw up. (It was the first time I'd thrown up since that summer day on the Mohican River.) I was hoping it would make me feel better, but it didn't. An hour later, I had to throw up again.

After that, I was finally able to go to sleep. The chills subsided, and my electric blanket was making me hot. The ibuprofen

I took worked on the sore muscles, and when I got up in the morning, I felt perfectly normal, and did my morning pushups without the struggle I was expecting. It reminded me of the days I could sleep off the flu or a hangover in one night. Back when I was, you know...younger.

While I was at work, Patty spent the day cleaning the house. It looked great when I got home. One of our resolutions is to stop getting our dinners at fast-food restaurants, but Patty didn't want to cook after the housework all day, and she reminded me that all the kids got Mcdonald's gift cards for Christmas, and tonight would be a great time to use them.

Wednesday, December 27, 2017

When I got home this afternoon, I heard Patty upstairs with Kyle in his room, demanding he get off his Xbox and clean up his room. I heard her order him down to the kitchen to get a trash bag. Since I was in the kitchen already, I thought I would do the boy a favor and bring a trash bag up to him. I did him a further favor by cutting off the Wi-Fi to his Xbox so he could clean his room without distraction. I thought I was being a very helpful dad.

Kyle didn't agree.

Thursday, December 28, 2017

When I got home today, Patty was cutting a pineapple that she bought at the grocery store. She likes to feed the kids fresh pineapple instead of junk food. The kids like pineapple, and so do I, but they like junk food, too. Kyle still sneaks food up into his bedroom, despite our threats to take away his Xbox.

I remember when *I* would sneak food, not up to my bedroom, but into my office or into my car or something like that. I can remember days when I would drop Patty off at Target and then go fill up the van with gas. And I would often stop at Taco Bell or Chick-fil-A and eat something quickly before I picked her up. I was selfish, and I didn't want to share. That seems like a lifetime ago now.

Friday, December 29, 2017

Patty has gained another pound, so she is at 218. She is mad at herself, and is making resolutions to log her food and eat more protein and do the treadmill and be more disciplined.

It's not like I can judge. I haven't been very good this week, eating a few Frostys from Wendy's. And I weigh myself tomorrow. So, I'm going to shut up.

Saturday, December 30, 2017

The scale was kind to me today. Even though I had a less-than-perfect week, I actually lost half a pound. I'll keep my log at 193, even though I'm a little bit less than that.

I went to work tonight, and it started to snow. And it didn't stop the whole time I was there. Driving was slow and treacherous, and the plows and salt trucks could not keep up. It was cold and getting colder, and after the weight loss, I am much more sensitive to the cold.

Meanwhile, Patty was home, on the couch in front of the fire, with a cup of English breakfast tea, complaining about Netflix being slow. She's watching Netflix, but *I'm* the one who's chilling. Literally.

Sunday, December 31, 2017

We're in a serious cold snap. I looked at the weather this morning, and it's going to be in the single digits for the next 10 days or so, sometimes dipping below zero. I hate this.

A few months after I started dating Patty in 1995, I had surgery on my hand and was off work for a couple of weeks. We had a similar cold snap and a snowstorm, and I was sitting in my studio apartment with nothing to do. So, I packed a bag, and called Patty at work to tell her that I'm driving down to Florida. She thought I was kidding, but I wasn't. She wanted me to wait for her to get off work so she could kiss me goodbye, but I wanted to leave while I had a few hours of daylight left. So I set out, and kept driving South. I stayed the night in a roadside motel in Georgia, and the following day I was in Key West.

I reminded her about that this morning, and told her, "Let's just go. Forget work and school. Let's get out of this cold. It will be an adventure!"

Once again, she thought I was kidding. She knows I wouldn't dare go without her this time. And she's right. But, it's tempting...

We were home this New Year's Eve. While watching the ball drop on TV, I hugged Patty hard, and thanked her for this amazing year. And I *really* meant it. As the kids shouted a countdown to zero, the last thing I saw before I gave her our traditional midnight kiss was her smile, and a reflection of the living room fire dancing in her moistening eyes.

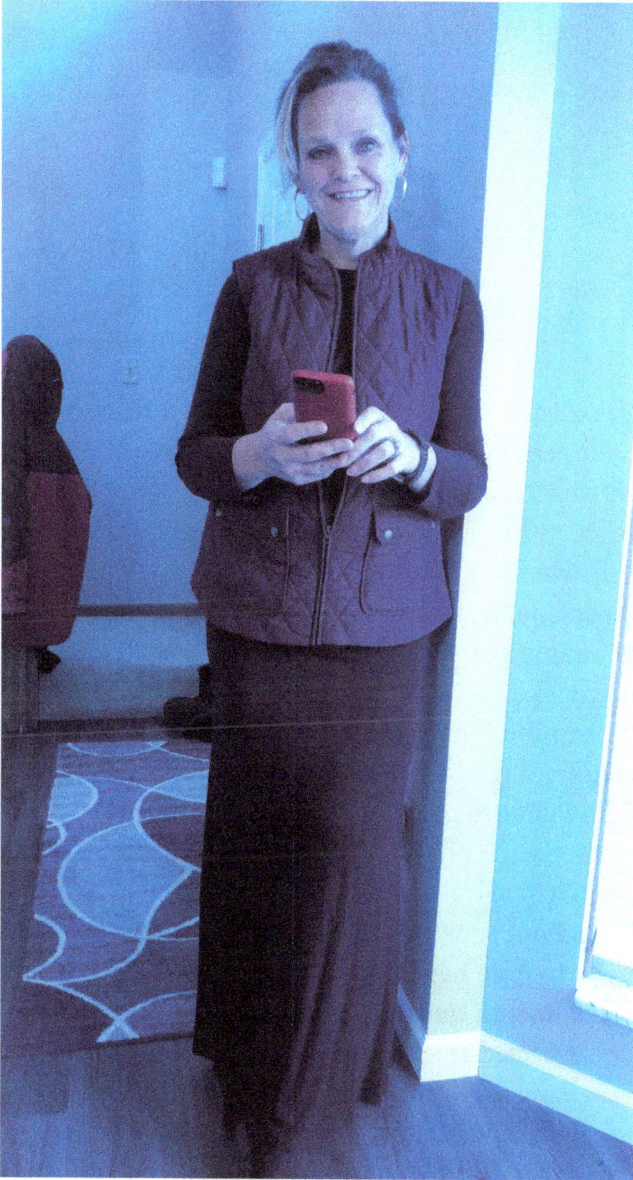

Patty after a 100+ pound weight loss.
January 2018. 400 days after surgery.

EPILOGUE

I predicted that Patty would become a new woman, and she certainly has. She is in her late forties, and she is tall, slender, elegant, and confident. I tease her sometimes, by saying she looks like a college professor, or a TV anchorwoman, especially when she wears her glasses. She sometimes still has a bubbly personality, which she honed well to compensate for her heavyset frame, but she strikes a much different image now. She looks more like a woman to be respected, to be taken seriously. She has admitted that people *do* seem to treat her with more respect now. She is more assertive, like I thought she would be. She is less willing to put up with the guff that people have dished out before. She has fundamentally changed. And that means I still need to change along with her.

Throughout most of our years of dating, courtship, and marriage, my role has been like a river pilot. That's a seaman who specializes in guiding a large, oceangoing vessel along a narrow, restricted river. It's a skill that takes years to develop. There are dangers around every bend. Shoals, sandbars, waterfront seawalls, and shifting water levels that threaten to run a ship aground, causing delays, or even damage. I've helped Patty navigate a river throughout the course of our relationship. I knew her size was a problem for her health, and her self-esteem, but I was determined that our relationship be a safe place for her to be herself. I've *never* criticized her weight; I've always called her beautiful, and I meant it. I've fixed broken furniture, I've massaged her aching muscles, I've supported her through dieting attempts and doctor appointments and emergency room visits. I've injected her with insulin every day when she had gestational diabetes during her first pregnancy. I've helped her avoid obstacles to her happiness, and tried my best to keep her in the channel. Over those couple of decades, I've become a pretty decent river pilot.

But this past year has presented me with a new challenge. The narrow, dangerous river that kept Patty restricted has widened. She can smell the salt in the air. She can hear the cry of the gulls. Before long, Patty will enter open water, slicing through the ocean swells at full throttle, like she was designed and built to do. She's about to enter a vast new world without limits. And, at that time, she will no longer need a river pilot.

She will need a sea captain.

This is a skill set I have not developed. It will mean change for me, too. I will have to become a new kind of husband, one who can handle her new energy and her pursuit of new opportunities. She will define happiness differently, and I have to be willing and able to adapt. Patty has lost over 100 pounds, and in doing so, she has a new ocean of potential. She has slain her dragon, the one that has kept her in chains for so, so long. If I'm going to be a worthy companion, I will have to learn to navigate this new phase of our marriage. I will have to draw strength from places I may not have.

Fortunately, I have earned some new strength, too. I made that decision on surgery day to change with her. I've lost 100 pounds, as well. I've sworn off the garbage food I used to love. I've gotten leaner, and stronger, and more capable. I've developed new habits, new strength, and a new outlook. And along the way, I've earned Patty's confidence. I've earned her trust. I've earned her respect. We're both cruising blindly into a future that we could not have predicted, and I might not be the perfect man to accompany her into it.

But she knows I have promised her that I will try my level best. And that promise has some past performance backing it up. And that, that opportunity to become her sea captain, is the greatest gift Patty has given me.

Spring/Summer 2018

Starting in January, I began slacking off in journaling. I found I was just repeating myself, and was unable to find new and interesting things to write about. We were eating pretty much the same things day to day, and we've settled into a routine. We both plateaued in our weight, and we both gained a few pounds, then lost them again. Patty is hovering between 200 and 210, and I am hovering between 190 and 200. I still do my pushups and pullups on alternate days, and I try to walk Maverick or do the treadmill three days a week.

My doctor calls me a "poster child" for how to respond to a diabetes diagnosis, and he told me on my most recent visit that I don't have the disease anymore. He told me I could still *get* it, if I returned to the old habits that caused it in the first place, but if I were seeing him for the first time today, he would neither diagnose it nor treat it.

Patty still has periodic followup appointments with her bariatric surgeon, but he says he is very pleased with her progress. One day, I hope she will be pleased with it as well.

We only took that one dancing lesson, and afterwards, Patty didn't want to do it anymore. She complained of foot pain and dizziness. I decided to give that up. Maybe after the kids are older, and if *they* can persuade her, she might do it. But I really want to find an activity we can do together, one that we both enjoy. Maybe, skydiving?

Throughout the winter and spring of 2018, Patty's mom continued to go in and out of the hospital due to her breathing problems. Patty continued to be her advocate, visiting her daily, and pressing her medical team to give her mother the best care they could.

In April, Patty, the kids, and I took a trip to the North Carolina coast to attend the wedding of my niece, Sara, on the beach. It was a beautiful spring weekend, and Patty and Kaitlyn were included in the group of ladies from the wedding party that had their hair and makeup done at a local salon. Patty was gorgeous in her aqua-blue floral gown and her light white jacket. She received so many compliments on her weight loss, she didn't want to return home after the week was over. The groom, a real-estate photographer, had someone flying a drone over the beach during the wedding, and Patty told me she was annoyed by the noise the drone was making. But it helped create an amazing wedding video, which is on Vimeo and entitled *Kahuna Wedding.*

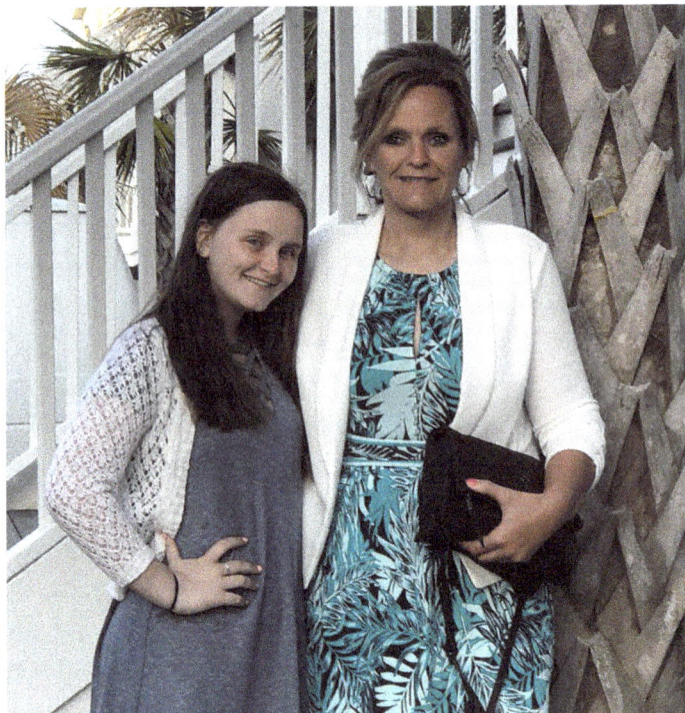

*Kaitlyn & Patty at Sara & Andrew's beach wedding
in North Carolina*

In early June, not long after we returned to Ohio, Patty's mom was admitted to the hospital for the last time. After a days-long vigil, she took her final breath, surrounded by her four daughters and her husband of fifty years, Bill. Her funeral was beautiful, and was attended by many dozens of the people who loved her.

The grieving process is arduous, and the family is still going through it. Patty still often finds herself, out of habit, picking up the phone to call her mom. Spring has brought cardinals back to Ohio, and occasionally one will be spotted in our back-yard by Kaitlyn. She sees the bright red bird as a sign from her

Grandma, a sign that she is happy and untroubled, and wants Kaitlyn not to worry. Patty reminds her, "there are no strokes in Heaven."

For our 18th anniversary in September, I took my bride to another concert, much like the one I recounted at the beginning of this book. Back then, we saw Amy Grant, and struggled in our seats. This time, we saw Adam Levine and Maroon 5. Music has changed a lot in the past twenty years. Popular music has become less melodic, and more of a "track and hook" style.

But it hasn't changed as much as Patty and I have. The seats were no longer a physical and emotional encumbrance. We enjoyed the event so much more. We danced in the aisle. We fit in with everybody else. We felt young, and alive again. What we've done together is something that no one can ever take away.

"In the beginning, I created a journal. In the end, it created me." I started this journal as a tool. I knew this would be the most consequential year of our marriage, and I knew I would forget so many valuable details if I didn't write them down. I was using it to keep myself accountable; to urge myself to keep at it, every day, even those days when every bone in my sore body wanted to give up. I wasn't sure if it would work, but to my surprise, it did.

And over the weeks and months, it became a story, one I could refer back to, and one that will hopefully keep me from backsliding. But even here at the end, Patty still doesn't know a thing about it. And that is about to change.

My plan is to bundle these pages all up, add a few photos, design a book cover, and publish it. I'm going to publish one book. One sole, singular copy. I'm going to gift-wrap it and add a sappy card. And then, I'm going to hand it to Patty.

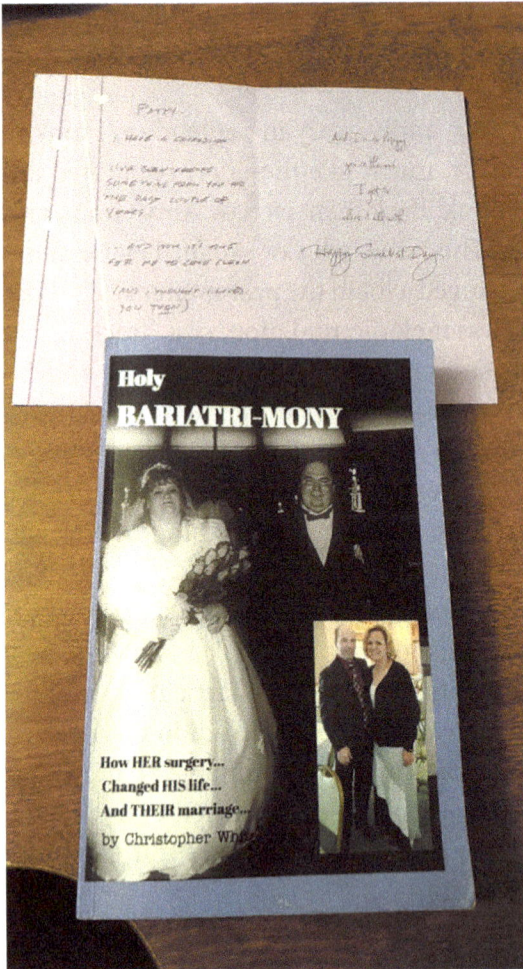

October 2018: The single draft copy of the book that Chris gave to Patty as a gift. The card reads, "Patty-I have a confession. I've been keeping something from you for the past couple of years...and now it's time for me to come clean. (And I thought I loved you then.)
Christopher

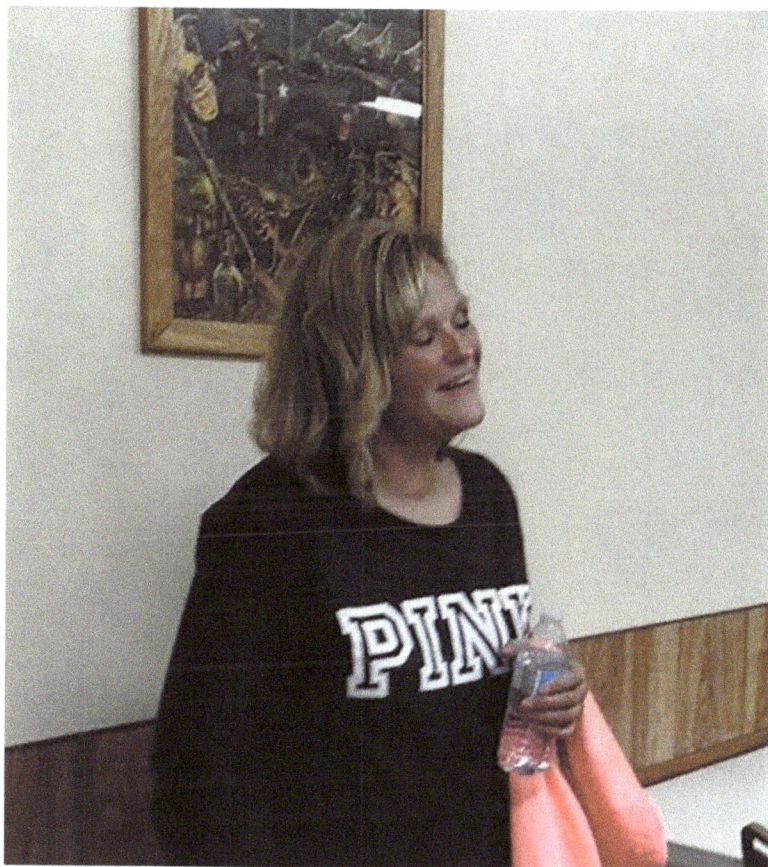

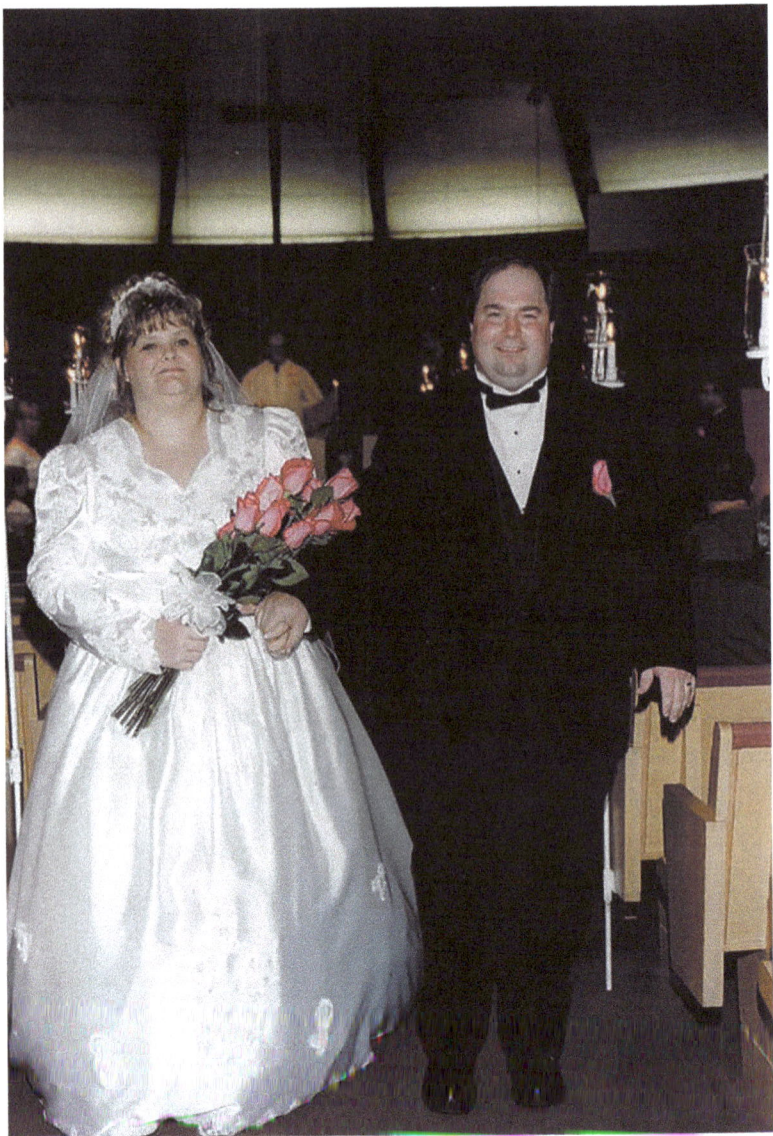

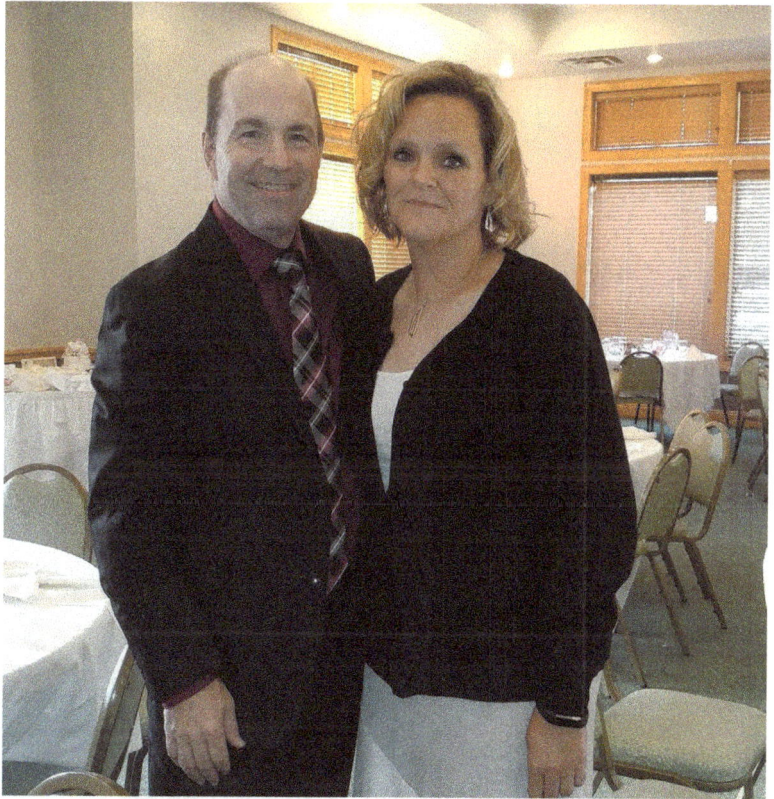

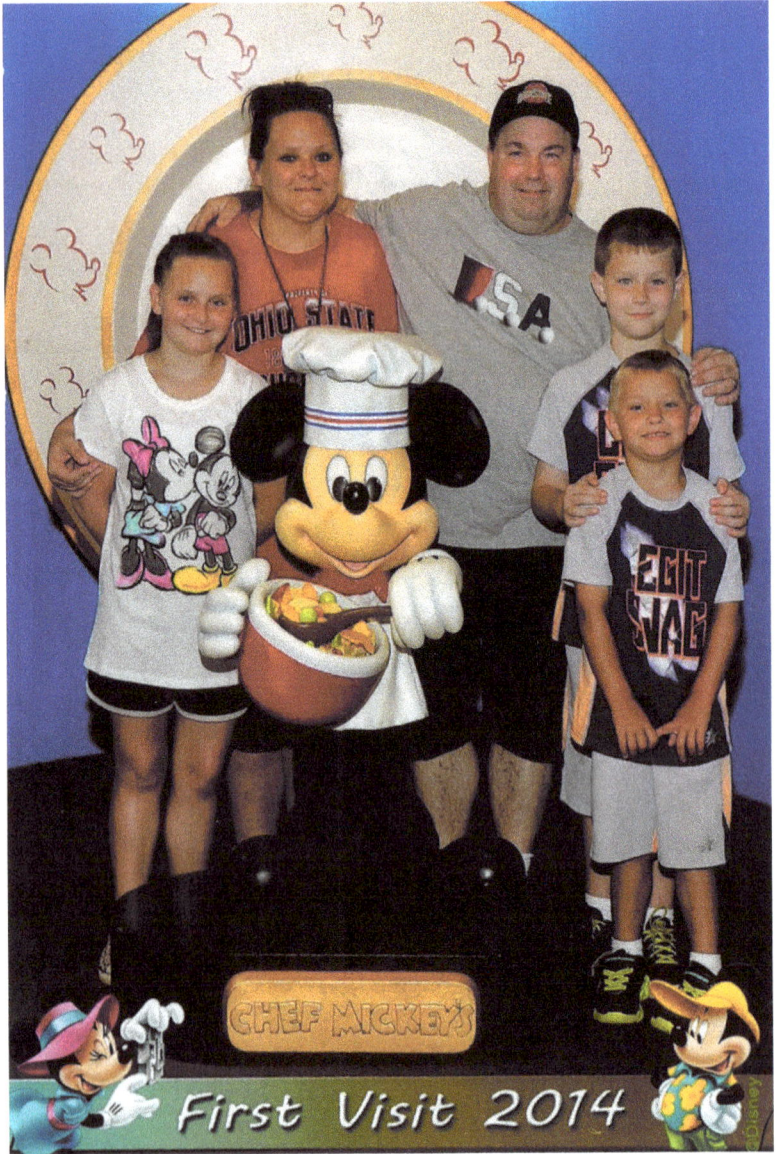
CHEF MICKEY'S

First Visit 2014

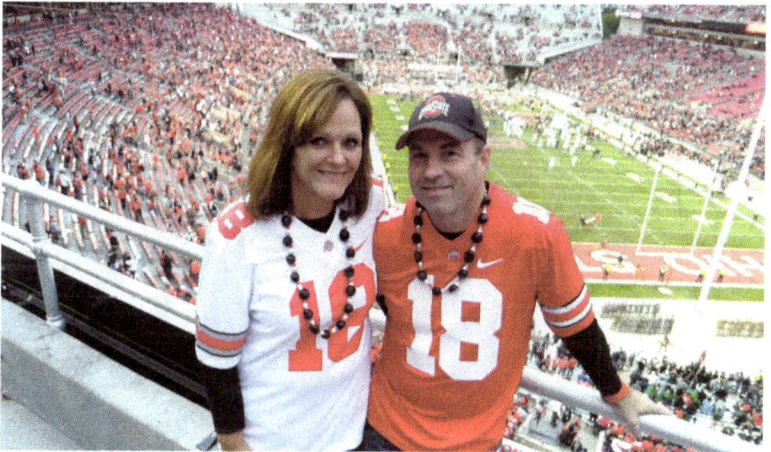

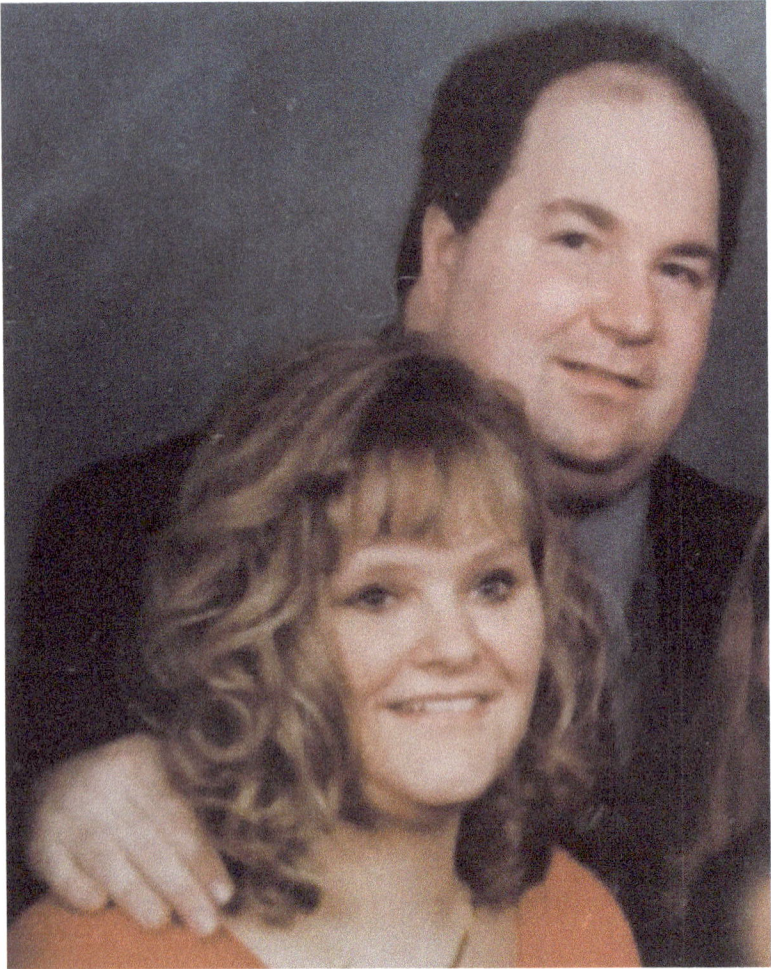

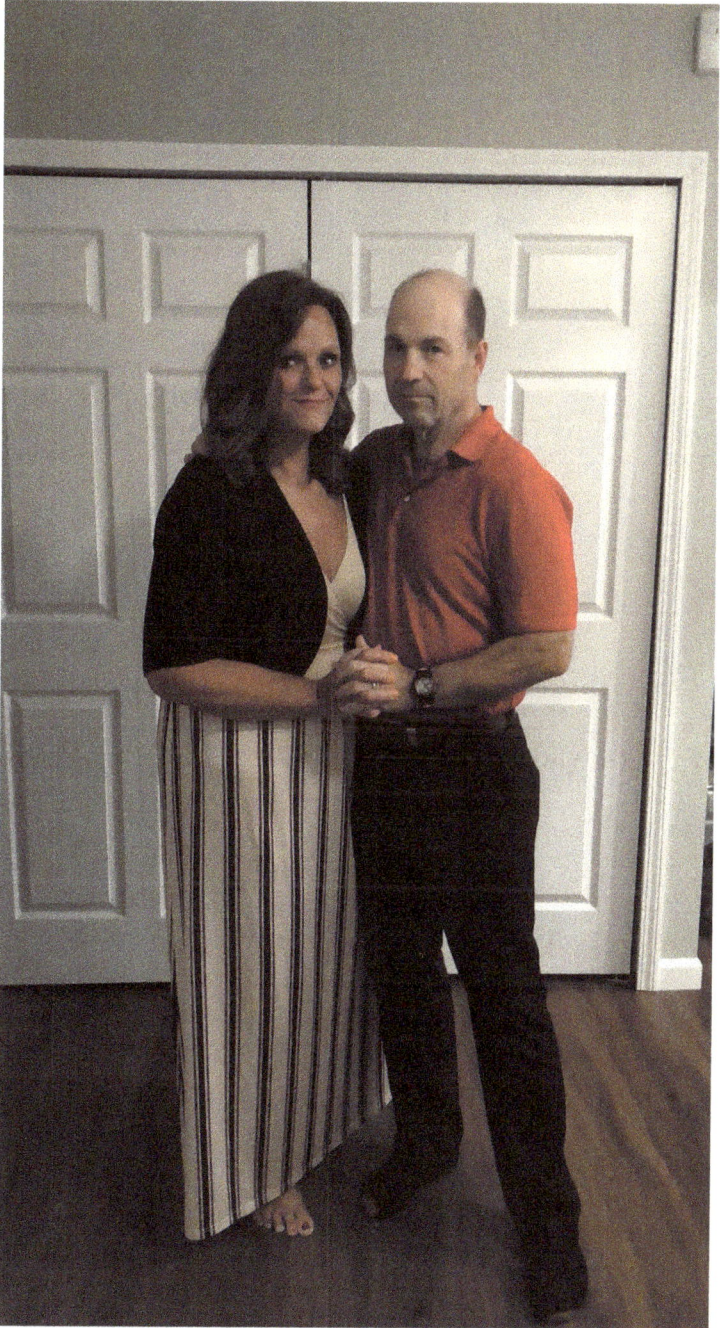

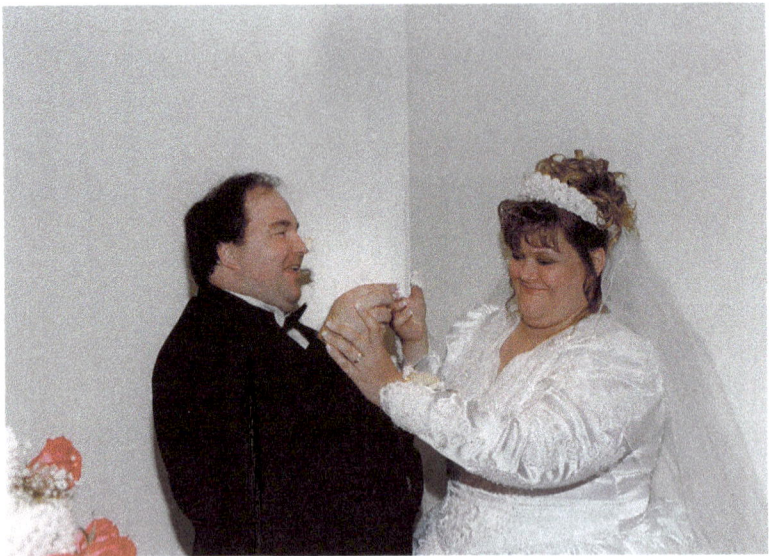

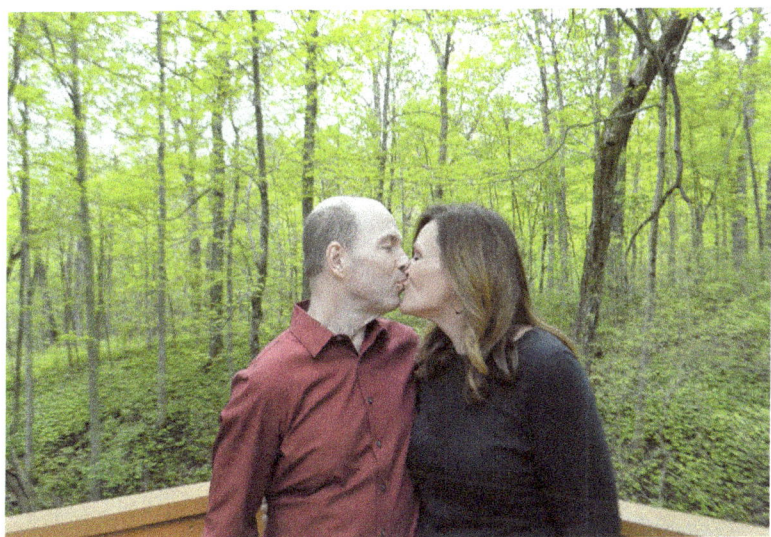

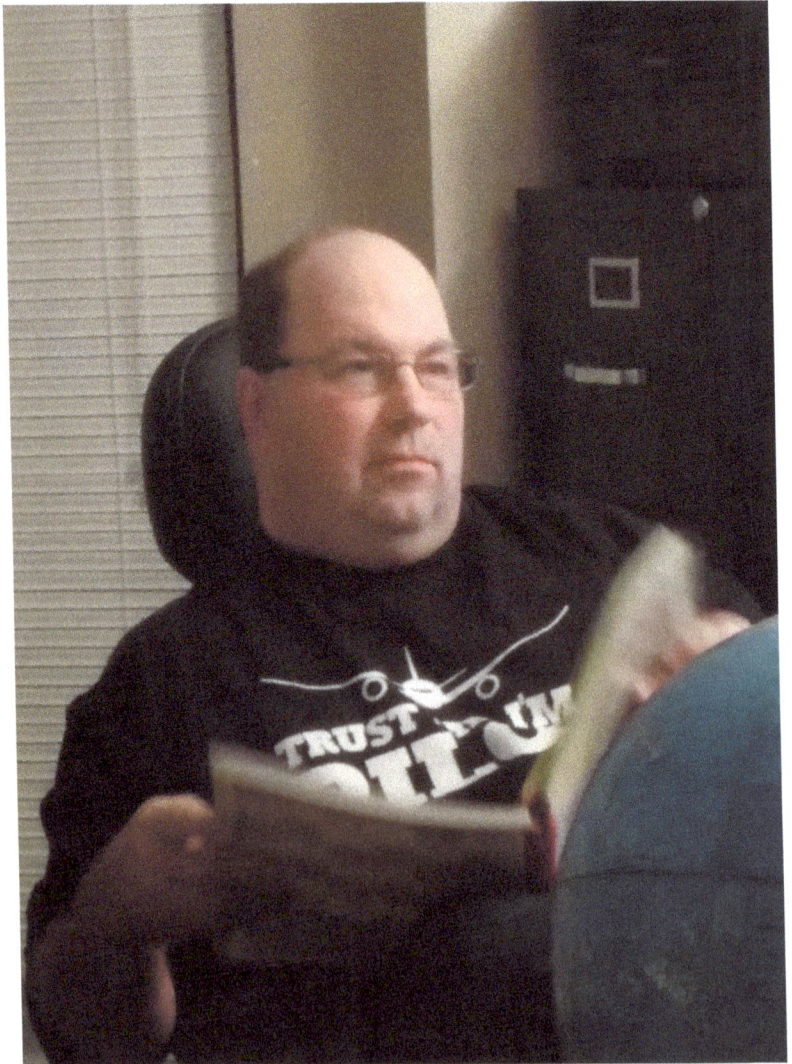

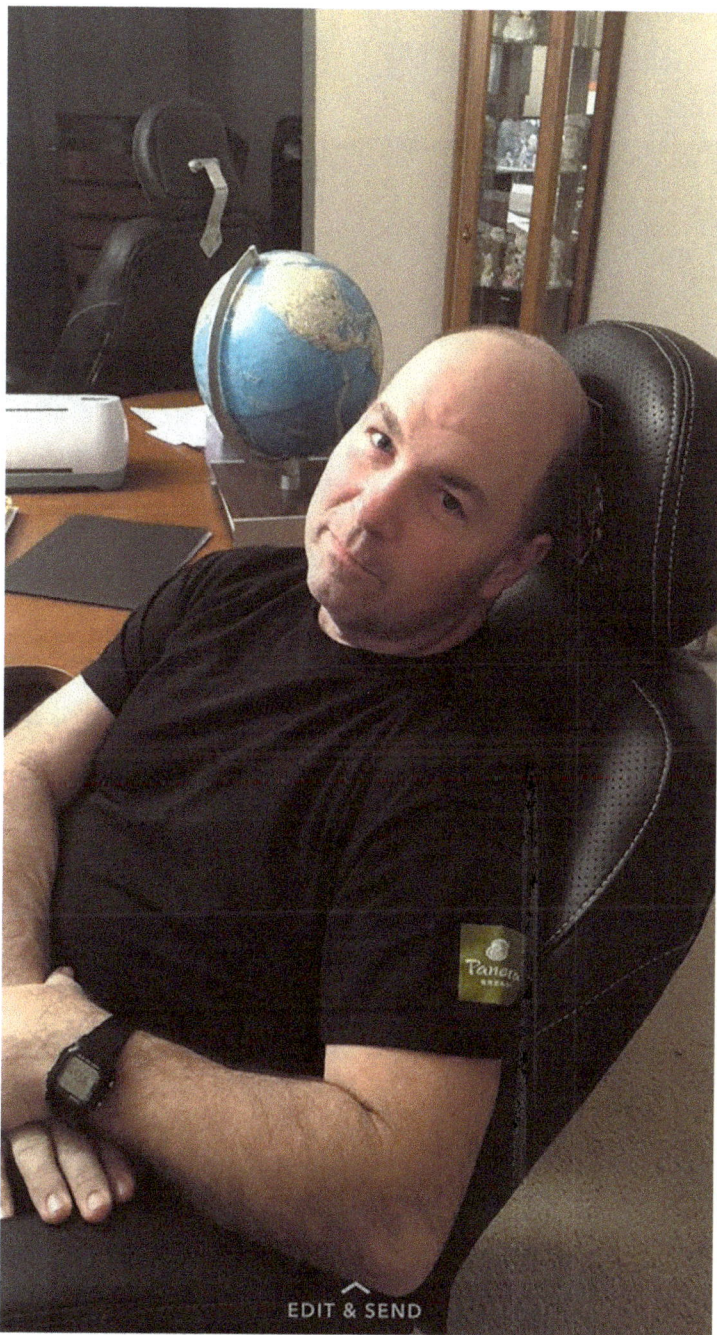

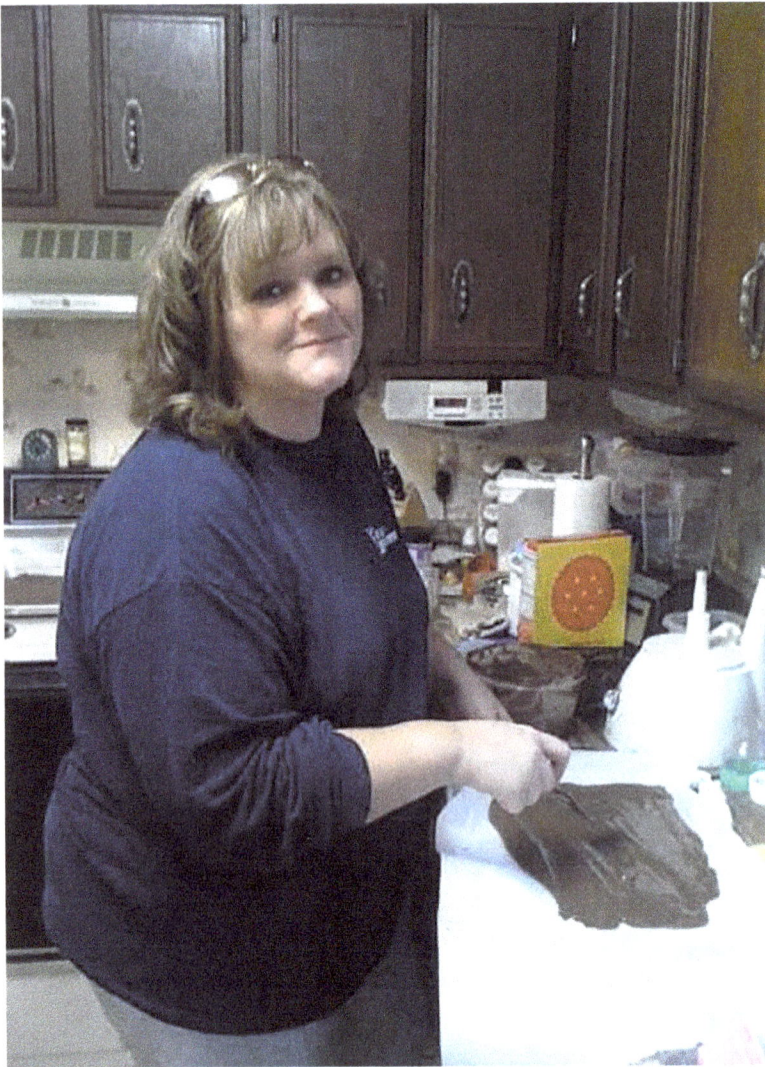

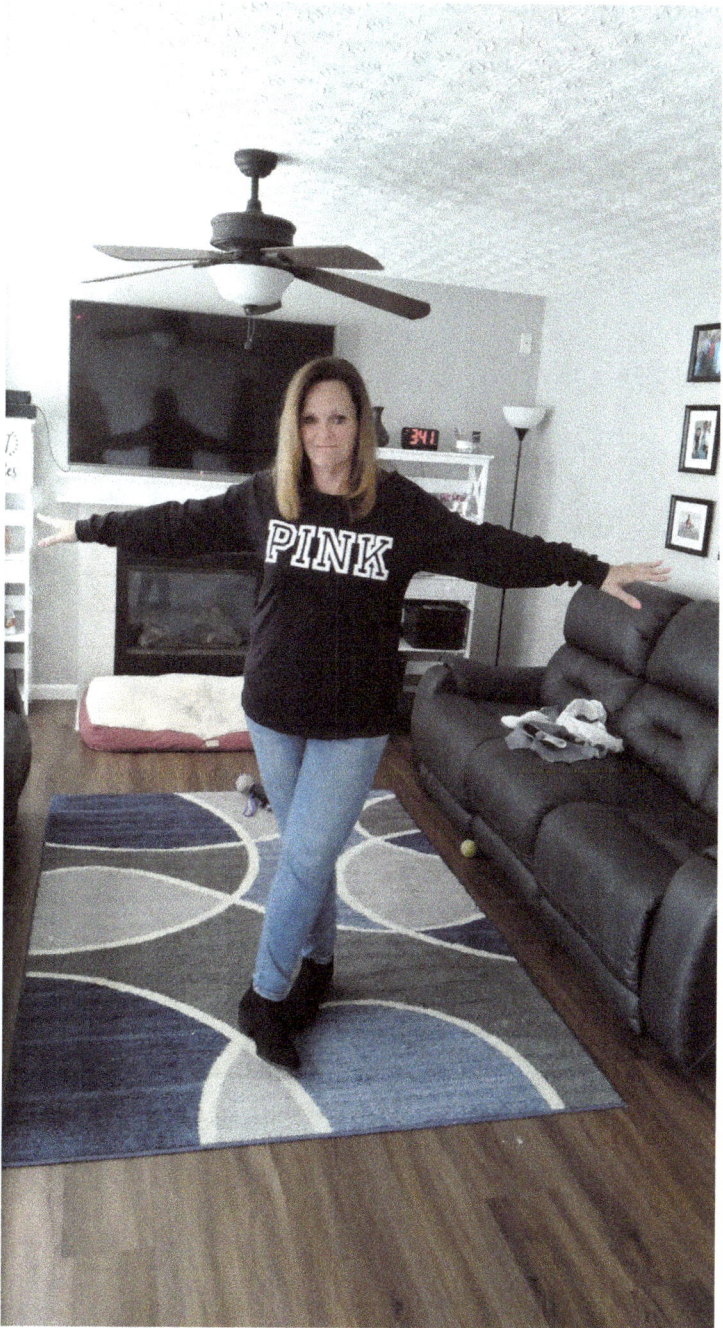

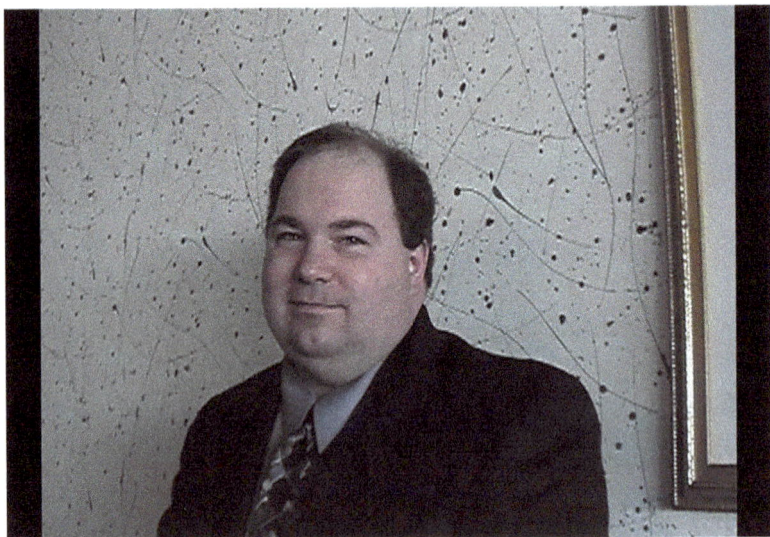
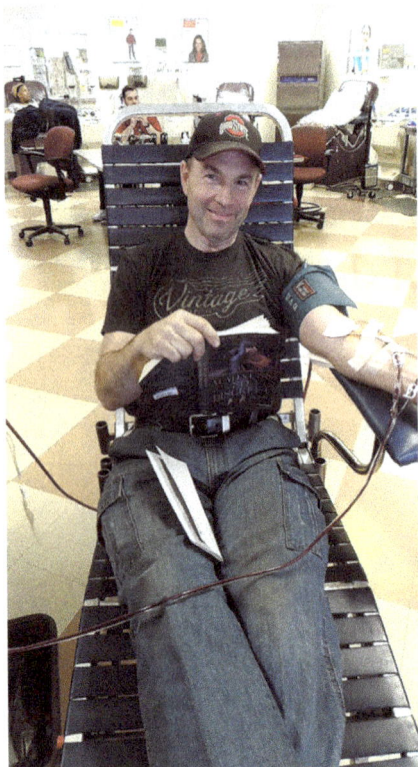

PATTY'S CHAPTER

*U*p, down, up, down, up, down......I'm sure everyone with weight issues knows this cycle all too well. I've had a weight problem my whole life. I started getting heavy about the age of thirteen. I got made fun of at school, and on the bus, and even by some of my loved ones. I was called names like two ton tessie and fatso. At school, there was one girl in particular that always made fun of me by saying I had 'elephantitis' and of course, others would follow. On the school bus some days people would sing "Fatty Patty two by four can't fit through the bathroom door". It never ended and today all that would be considered bullying. I had an uncle walk up the stairs behind me at a Christmas gathering and he told his daughter, "if you eat that you'll look like her". I heard but pretended I didn't. I wasn't happy, but I put on the prettiest face and pretended my life was good. I felt I had no escape, so I turned to food more and more. Every year I got heavier and I was making things worse because I was feeding my emotions.

In high school, if I ever said I had a crush on someone, they'd joke and say "he'll never date you, have you looked in the mirror lately?" I had a boyfriend in high school. I even attended church with him. Very nice guy; he must have been brave to date the "fat girl". I was shy when it came to dating since I was always told no guy would ever date me. I felt special, he was a senior and I was a freshmen. Eventually things ended, after he went to college and I was probably a little too immature and not experienced with dating and very unsure of myself. He found a new girlfriend. She was thin and the only thing that I could think of again--I'm too fat, worthless and I'll never find anyone. As I got older, I was not comfortable around people. I hung out mostly at home, with my mom or with my best friend. I started feeling worthless, that I would never amount to anything, or be good enough. I carried this all into my adult life. I feel as though I didn't accomplish my potential because, how could I when the people closest to me were calling me names?

I decided if this was who I was going to be I better get used to it and make the best of my life. I dated a few other guys until I found my prince charming in August of 1995. On that day I stopped by my sister's work to drop something off. Later that night she told me a guy there thinks I'm pretty, and he would ask me out, but he wanted to pay off his car loan first. I was curious, so I started going by and finally met this guy. His name was Chris. I really liked him too. He was cute and seemed super nice. He definitely had it together. I eventually asked *him* out (the fat girl came out of her shell). He came over to my house to watch a movie and the night ended with a kiss that said it all. I knew from that moment he was "the one". I was going to marry this guy. I told my mom this and I knew she thought I was crazy, but she just smiled and said ok. Chris didn't make this easy. In fact, he told me he wasn't ever getting married or having children. He was serious and I looked at him and said we'll see. We dated three years, became engaged and he started graduate school. He said he couldn't get married until he graduated and I was ok with that. We got married September 15, 2000.

I started a job with a great company and not quite a year into working there I developed some autoimmune diseases. I first lost lower vision in my right eye then lost it all in that eye except some peripheral vision. It then moved to the lower half of my left eye. The doctor that saw me said it was because of the spots on my lungs called sarcoidosis. I had to see several specialists. I ended up having to leave my job since I was an IT analyst and working on the computer 8-9 hours a day was not working anymore, because my eyes were swelling shut.

I wanted to become a mom. I was worried about my diseases and my weight, and I tried dieting over and over again. I'd lose a little and then gain it back plus more. I was well over 300 pounds at this point and kept getting told by my doctors that I needed to lose weight.

In December 2002, we found out I was pregnant (after a miscarriage that previous summer). I was so excited and nervous at the same time. I developed gestational diabetes and started measuring my blood sugars and gave myself insulin. It was a pain. However, I did manage to lose weight with this pregnancy and I remember weighing around 267 when our daughter was born in September 2003.

Again, more diets and more weight gain but I did go on to have two more children (both boys). One in July of 2005 and one in December of 2007. I ended up being diagnosed with several more autoimmune diseases and also survived thyroid cancer. One thing all the doctors and specialists could agree on—*Patient is morbidly obese.* I was not a typical overweight person since I didn't have hypertension, joint issues, diabetes or high cholesterol.

My kids were getting older and starting school and one of my biggest fears is that I would embarrass them or they would get made fun of because of their mom's size. As they got older, the kids got mean. I babysat a boy that was 9 at the time and I went out to our pool. He told my son, watch out if she gets in; all the water is going out! I acted like I didn't hear him, but the fact of the matter is I did. I felt horrible, but I knew this was bound to happen.

In 2014, I attended a seminar on bariatric surgery. I loved listening to the success stories, but I was scared of what they had to do. They would take my stomach (after making my stomach half its size) and attach it to the lower half of the small intestine. It is completed by connecting the top portion of the divided small intestine to the small intestine further down so that the stomach acids and digestive enzymes from the bypassed stomach and first portion of the small intestine will eventually mix with the food. The surgeon talked about how important taking your vitamins and adhering to the dietary guidelines would be after this surgery. I went away really thinking about it, but I wasn't 100% sure that was the answer for me.

The following year, I attended two more seminars. One in the winter and one in the spring. I knew I wanted to do something and I loved the success stories. The seminar in the spring had a surgeon by the name of Dr. Thomas Sonnanstine. I really loved how passionate he was about what he was doing. He said there was also another procedure called the gastric sleeve. I listened very carefully. This didn't seem to be as involved and the complications seemed to be even less. At this point, I found the surgery I wanted to try. He did stress that it's not a magic pill; that it's only a tool--*You* still have to do the work. I talked to him afterwards and told him what I was thinking. I told him I weighed about 347 pounds and that I have tried so many diets but I didn't have any health issues *yet* related to my weight. I told him I was interested in the sleeve and he agreed I'd be a great candidate. I proceeded with all the paperwork and started the nutrition counseling and all the tests that were required. About 6-9 months later, I would be having my surgery after a long struggle with the insurance company to approve this. It was a difficult road considering the only criteria I actually met was my BMI. I was denied first and then after I pursued it further, I finally got my approval! November 29, 2016 would be the start of the new me and I couldn't be happier. Sure I was nervous, but I was also ready to lose this weight that was keeping me from living my life.

I was also nervous about my marriage. Would I change so much my husband would hate me? I sure have been reading the stories and one day I looked at my husband and told him how I felt and he said it'll be ok. I'm not really sure what he meant but I do know he was reading bariatric stories and would talk to me about them. I've never been thin and I've never had guys pursue me, so how would I deal with this? Everyone told me I was pretty and I'd even been asked why are you hiding your beauty behind all that fat? If you'd only lose weight, you'd feel better.

When I was in the pre-op holding area, I had a panic attack. I spoke with my dad on the phone before I left for the hospital and he told me he'd support me if I didn't go through with this surgery. He said you're big boned and he'll do whatever he can to help me. I had been having dreams of dying the whole week before. However, I had already made this decision and I was going to go through with it. When my surgeon met with me before the surgery, I asked him if I was going to die. He said he can't promise that, but he thought I'd do great. He asked if I was having second thoughts and I told him no. I asked if they could give me something in my IV to relax me and they did. I'm so glad I didn't allow that scared, broken woman to make my decision that day.

After surgery, I had gas pain pretty bad. The nurses gave me pain meds and I slept a lot the first night. When I woke up, I felt better and explained my pain and they told me it was probably just gas and the best way to deal with this is to get up and walk. So I did. They were so impressed that I was in the hall all the time. We even turned this into a game and they showed me the dry erase board and told me to mark each time I went for a walk. I wanted to feel better and I wanted to do everything the doctor said. I did not take any pain meds the rest of the time I was in the hospital. I didn't need them. I'm usually a wimp with pain, but to be honest I wasn't having any. I do remember the surgeon coming in the next morning and when he saw me he told me I looked great and he would've never guessed I'd been through surgery. He was very impressed. I also want to say, things are better when you have a great support system. My mom, dad, mother-in-law, husband and best friend were there. My best friend (Jen) who has her own family even stayed an entire day and well into the night and walked around the halls with me. This is what matters and this will help you succeed.

Two days after surgery, I finally got to go home. Oh, the thought of finally sleeping in my own bed! And boy, did I sleep. After getting into a new way of eating and trying to figure out what to eat and how much, things were great. But, it wasn't always that way. I had times I was so angry for doing this and kept questioning myself, why? When I started seeing the weight loss and people started noticing, it made it worth it. I just had to get over the first 3-4 months and I would be fine, I just wish someone would've told me this. I will also admit, my journey was definitely made easier because my husband was dieting and I wasn't dealing with him eating pizza, cake, cookies or a lot of fast food. We had started adopting a healthy lifestyle and having him by my side made it *so* much easier.

I was a slow loser. I'm not sure why, but I felt horrible when I would go to the doctor and he expected 10 pounds and I'd lose 5 pounds. I totally understand why people don't go to the doctor when they're overweight--the scales! I always thought I'd have better and faster results but I got what I got and today I'm so much better off. My surgeon always encouraged me and I tried hard not to let him down. He was always optimistic and it made me want to try harder. By the end of my second year, I had lost 109 pounds. My starting weight the day of surgery was 317 pounds and I weighed 208 pounds at the end of my second year.

I went through the biggest loss of my life June 14, 2018...I lost my mom. She was my biggest cheerleader and my best friend. She supported me always. She was 70 years old and I sat by her bedside when she took her last breath. I gained some weight. I went from 208 to 215 in 6 months. I was mad at myself, because I went back to my emotional eating. Today, I hang out around 210-215. I really wish I could lose the other 40 pounds, and I will. I have the tools; I just have to use them.

I chose not to tell anyone about my surgery. I had been getting so many compliments and people looking twice. My daughter was a cheerleader and her friends asked her one day where her mom was and she pointed to me. They told her they didn't see me. She swore to them it was me and she had to walk up to me and point me out. Their mouths dropped, they told me I looked great. That made my day, and I'm sure it made hers. I wasn't into pictures most of my life, but my daughter is always taking my picture. I guess I should appreciate the fact that she does, I don't really have a lot of pictures before when my kids were little and it breaks my heart. I'm still unsure about unleashing my secret, but it is what I did and I'm now a better mom and wife because of it. There are some people that know and others that still don't but when it comes out maybe I can help someone. I'm not perfect, but I try and I have maintained my weight for almost 3 years. It's not a quick or easy fix, but I chose it because I felt it's what I needed. Are there any regrets, NO. Do I like myself better, YES. Do I still criticize myself, YES. One of the biggest issues I have is all the loose skin. I try to hide it, but it's not always easy. I still have moments I hate how I look. I need to develop a positive attitude and be happy. I have come a long way. Would I do it all again, YES. Do I still see the fat girl I used to be, YES, but not as often. After bariatric surgery there are NSV (non-scale victories) that people celebrate, and let me tell you if I concentrated on those instead of the scale, I'd be so happy. I'm finally living my life. I used to hide from things like concerts. I hated the thought of not being able to fit into the seats. I wouldn't go on plane rides for fear I'd have to ask for a seatbelt extension and I definitely would take up my seat plus some of the next. Now, I fly more than ever and walk down the aisle straight and not sideways bumping every person and getting horrible looks and I even have extra length on my standard seatbelt. I used to hate to go to the beach. Now, I'll go. I am still self conscious about the loose skin and stretch marks, but I need to accept this is who I am and I have accomplished a lot. Amusement Parks, never. I hated the walk, the rides and the looks fat people get. Now, I actually get on rides with my kids and totally enjoy them and especially love that I'm making them happy doing it. So many things have changed.

I have actually gone from shopping in "fat" stores to being able to go into any store and buy clothes. One day, I went into

Victoria's Secret/Pink and tried on bras. They actually fit and I broke down and cried. I could also wear their clothes, some in size medium but mostly large. I also went into American Eagle and was able to purchase a pair of jeans right off the shelf in a size 14. The joy my heart felt, I can't even explain. From my largest size 28 jeans and a 3X shirt going to a size 14 jeans and medium/large shirts--this is such a big deal and I needed to apologize ahead of time to my husband because I found a new joy for clothes shopping.

Would I ever offer advice to someone considering this surgery? YES, if they asked. My advice would be to remember this is a journey, not a race. It is not easy and you have to push through. But once you can eat solid food, you'll get into a routine and then it won't be as bad as you thought. You have to be committed and have a great support system. There are a lot of groups online if you don't have anyone or just want ideas or to vent. I'd also tell them to make sure they are ready. For a lot of us, we've hit our breaking point and there is always a reason we should lose weight. For me, I just didn't want to pass on an eating disorder, food obsession or body shame to my children so I had to get a handle on it before it got a bigger handle on me. I also wondered how I could be so successful at most things I do or try but I couldn't get control of my relationship with food. I was missing out on living, my life was always on hold waiting for me to be comfortable in my own skin.

But please be aware, I am not telling everyone that this is for them. I am telling you my story and how I decided that this is what I needed to do. I also took a long time in coming to this decision, it is a personal choice. Am I comfortable in my skin now? Not exactly, but I'm in a better place than I have been in a long time and I definitely feel like I'm living my life. I never realized how much my weight was taking from my life.

We all must go for our goals. A setback doesn't mean you have to give up, you just have to try harder. Every little step counts! One of my favorite quotes is "If you're going to quit anything, quit being lazy, quit making excuses and quit waiting for the right time". My right time started with Dr. Sonnanstine on November 29, 2016.

ABOUT THE AUTHOR

Christopher White is a tax preparer, bulk-paper courier, and a 30-year employee of Donatos Pizza. He lives and loves, works and writes in Columbus, Ohio.

www.ingramcontent.com/pod-product-compliance
Lightning Source LLC
Chambersburg PA
CBHW062115040426
42336CB00041B/986